PLANT-BASED
EATING

Penny Craig

Whole Food, High Protein, On-Budget Recipes, Hints for Keeping your Body's **pH** Alkaline, Boosting your Immune System, Strength, and Focus

bubbly&Co press

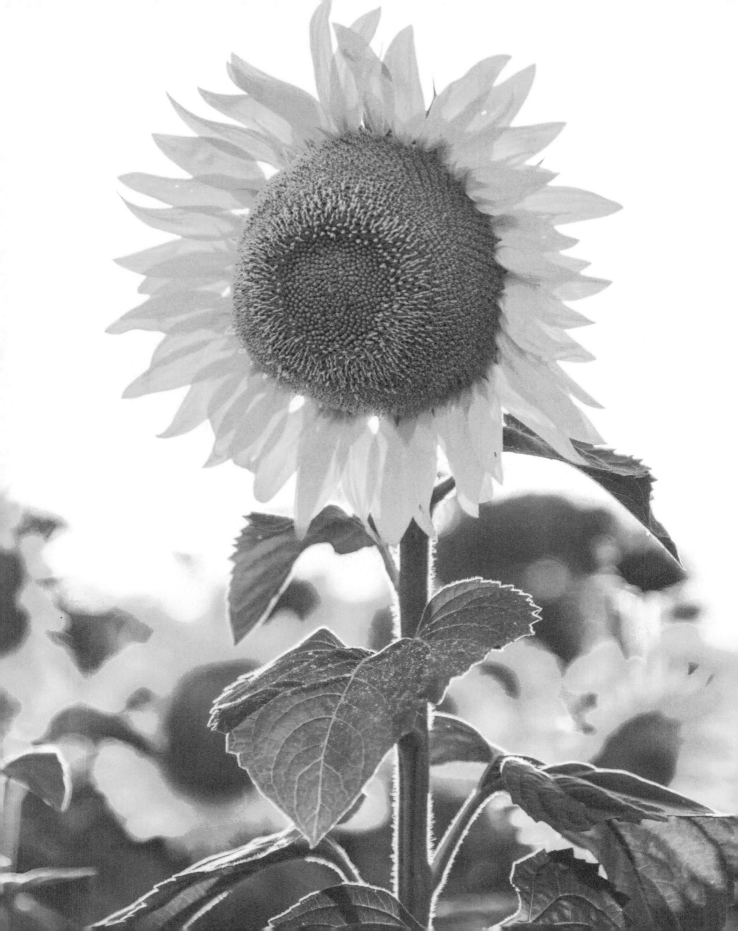

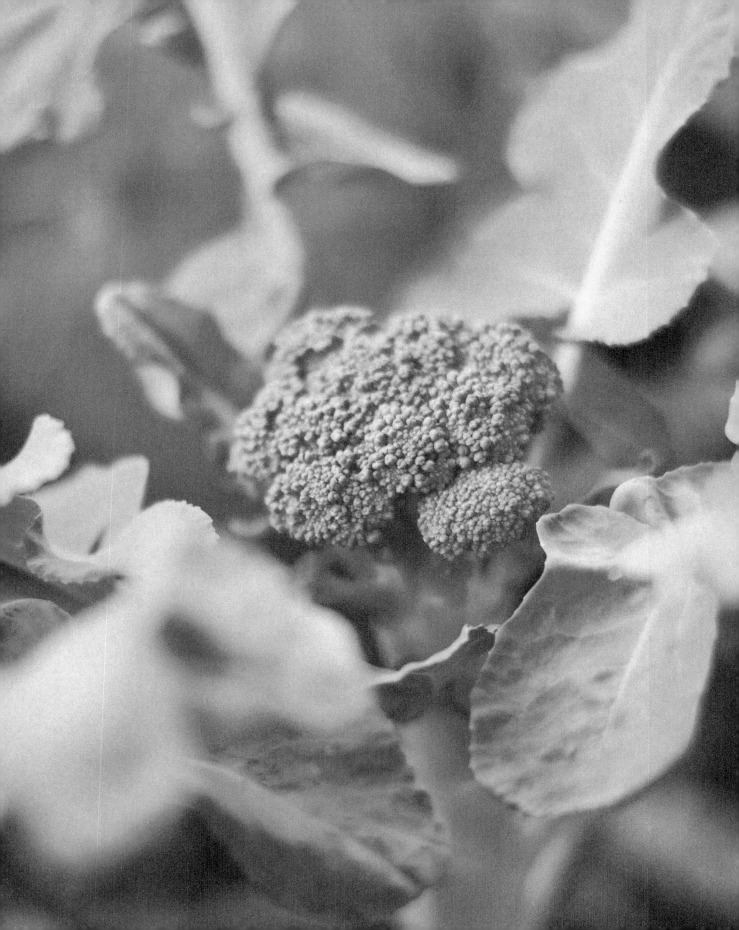

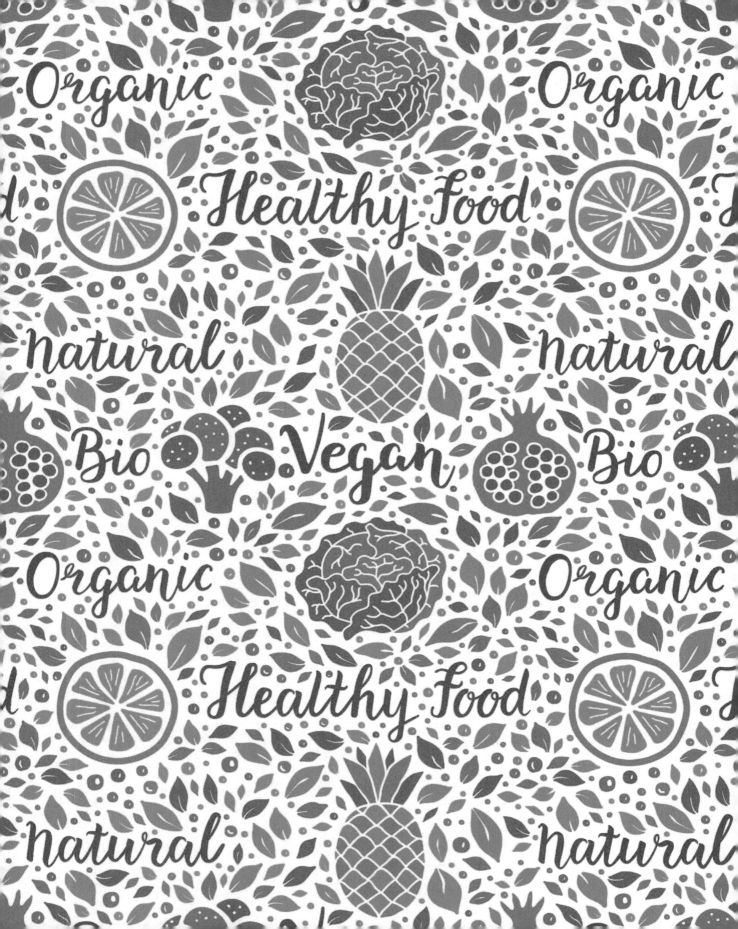

Introduction

Plant-based and whole food (PBWF) eating might sound like another simple diet for tree-huggers, or people who are a bit extreme and radical in their food choice, on the other hand it has grown, a wide folk movement really "falling in eat" with this way to nourish body&brain, basically because followers start to feel better, lighter, happier, brighter and detoxified, hereafter you may find many reasons and suggestions, ready to be absorbed, and put into daily practice.

The media-market has referred to plant-based food as the 'golden mean between vegetarianism and veganism because you can gain several benefits with less sacrifices...simply sayings, as... no pain no gain, or... seeing is believing...which do you prefer?

Substantially starting with the awareness that daily nourishment is our first **medicine**, should help us to cut back on wrong nutritional habits, for example the consumption of animal products, such as meat, dairy and processed foods have proven to be unhealthy and not budget friendly.

Recent scientific research has found that it is possible to gain extra weight, suffer from overall body inflammation, shortness of breath, bad moods and a foggy brain, when regularly eating animal-based and processed food. Reading food labels and tracing the manufacturing origin is always suggested during our daily shopping.

Increasing our own knowledge about healthy nutrition should be the aim. To be free from medications that we take to solve problems w**e** ourselves have created and lastly, avoid poisoning ourselves with junk food.

"Americans may live longer but sicker", behind this claim there is frightening and misleading understanding of the concept of prevention. For decades the cure was based on symptoms instead of on risk factors and causes, only recently the AHA (American Health Association) developed a list of correct behavior to follow and apply to prevent causes. New research report affirms that life expectancy in USA during the 21st century is lessening and the risk of millennials living less healthy and shorter lives than their parents, is real.

So, by switching to a PBWF diet you, can start, finally, to face, relief and solve several tedious and sticky health-troubles. Gaining information on the biological mechanisms and areas that regulate the human well-being is crucial, essential part of this information is Human' body's pH.

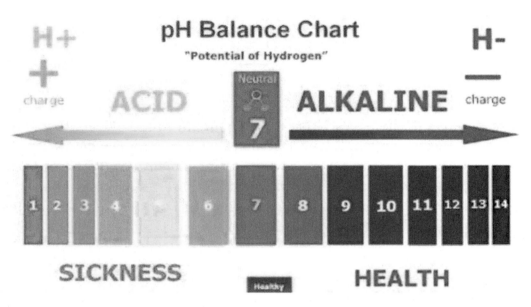

The **Alkaline pH** and **Acid pH** states balance in our body has such a profound influence on our health and well-being, it's hard to imagine. Some foods like lemon juice or vinegar will make the body more acidic while other foods like cucumbers or almonds will make our bodies more alkaline.

The consumption of alkaline food will help the human body, promoting better general health. Someone suffering from blood inflammation, arthritis, diabetes, cancer and other diseases may find that switching to an alkalized diet will significantly improve their general health and delay aging process.

When the body is more acidic than alkaline, it tends to attract several troublesome diseases, just like the ones mentioned above. Otherwise, alkalized bodies are less prone to diseases and are more energized, focused and positive on overall life goals.

People need to know a couple of things about acid and alkaline foods. Firstly, body fluids' pH is determined by many factors, such as our diets, lifestyle, stress levels...pH can be acidic or alkaline to the acidity or alkalinity of the water we drink, and the food we eat every day. Secondly, natural water is slightly alkaline, and we will notice the positive effect it has on our health. We all should keep ourselves hydrated, as much as possibly can, meaning we should drink the recommended amount of at least 2 liters daily consume.

What is the meaning of acid or alkaline body?

The concept of acid and alkaline consumption is based on balancing pH levels in the body. The most accurate way to know if your body is acidic or alkaline is through testing our saliva using pH test strips available online. However, there are also some ways to control if your body is more acidic than alkaline without having to test it every day.

Body' fluids are naturally slightly alkaline in general, but we need to maintain a balance between the acidic pH rate and the alkaline pH rate, so having an ideal pH level of 7-7,50, means everything is fine with feeding, drinking and training. Humans need to get better at checking pH rates frequently, at least twice a year, to know if their eating and lifestyle habits are in line with good health or if it is better to change something to create a better balance.

For example, if we mainly eat alkaline foods, our body will remain slightly alkaline overall and the opposite. But if we are consistently consuming acidic or alkaline foods for more than a month then the body will start to adjust to this change.

The best indicator of whether your body is acidic or alkaline is your health and well-being. If you have an acidic pH level, your health will tend to be poor, and you will feel tired most of the time. If you have an alkaline pH level, you will be healthier overall and feel very energetic, motivated and focused.

What makes PBWF eating so beneficial?

First, it helps, as just highlighted, to cure and reverse diseases, and become, energetic, motivated and focused. People who eat PBWF has lower cholesterol levels, are less likely to develop heart disease, and other chronic diseases. This type of lifestyle also make you lose weight, as it involves consuming a higher volume of fiber that will make you feel full for longer, that means in less snacking and bingeing during the day or night.

PBWF eating, is it easy on the budget?

A few easy rules need to be understood and to be put into practice on a daily basis. It will be worth finding out how a smart organization when shopping and cooking will help shape your new long-term well-being, saving your money and precious time to enjoy life's passions with loved ones and friends.

Increasing PBWF nourishment, will be the far-sighted way for us to decrease the ongoing destruction of our mother earth. It's estimated that animal intensive livestock farming contributes to approximately 30% of all greenhouse gas emissions.

This percentage is expected to reduce as more people opt for PBWF eating and eat much less meat and dairy products. As it stands, breeding an animal takes about **10 times** as much water and produces up to **100 times** as much waste and **CO2** compared to growing the same amount of food directly from seeds or plants.

Today **sustainability** is a very misused and raped word, without the understanding of its real meaning.

We must become sustainable first, for ourselves and our neighbors. Only after we have realized, understood and practiced this concept will we have the chance to contribute in an active way to the ambitious project of world sustainability. Once again, we need to make small changes in our daily lives that will subsequently be contributing towards the bigger changes to the world around us.

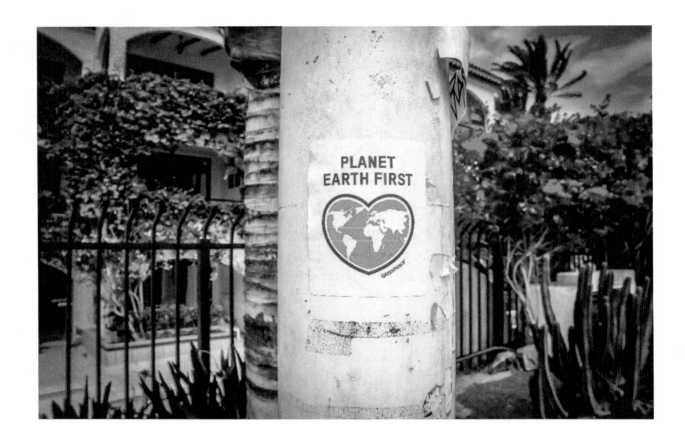

Chapter 1: Just Do Eat

Newbies to PBWF eating, or those who are just looking for a "working diet" that can preserve health, time and money, get ready to fall into this new beneficial journey. It is not a fad diet with crazy ingredients that sound good in theory, but you will never actually try. It is about simple, effective and resalable rules- recipes made from ethical family physicians-doctors and professional nutritionists that make better meals easy, fast and affordable while losing weight, improving your general wellbeing, helping also with a serious and dedicated daily work out plan.

Gut is the Key

"From the gut comes strut and where hunger reigns, strength abstains" Franciois Rabelais... Just to underline the importance of the gut in many human' life shades...Probably if you are reading, you are well willing to begin with a new chapter of your aware nutrition' life.

Statistics alert in USA, overweight and obesity are often associated with a higher risk of metabolic disorder, blood and joint inflammation, heart strokes, some kinds of cancer, diabetes type 2, skin diseases etc.
A wide number of Americans are very aware of the health limits of SWD or SAD (standard western-American diet), that is based on an animal and processed food diet. Obviously, this method leads to a dramatic increase of chronic diseases and unhealthy habits.

Food in the USA is the No. 1 cause of poor heath and premature death. Studies clearly report that a world switch to a plant-based & whole-food diet would have a massive impact on preventing an estimated 15 million adult deaths each year.

Evidence of nutrients source, determine gut wellbeing and consequent humans' longevity, who choose to follow a PBWF diet confirm a sudden positive change in digestion, a lighter feeling, better physical performance, significant changes in their general health, better mood and a sharper brain.

There are several ways that PBWF diets can improve general human well-being. Consuming a vegetable high-protein diet, makes it easier on the gut and also aids gut cleansing, which means becoming more active and building more awareness over time. You also experience less fatigue if you exercise. Less inflammation in the body due to the absence of junk food, more energy, clear head and feeling less sluggish every day.

Medical research and millions of trials around the world has shown that the consumption of a PBWF diet helps also to get less aggressive mood as opposed to animal based and processed food, it reduces, decreases and reverses pain-discomfort such as blood inflammation and arthritis. PBWF will make you feel confident, stronger and more stable, in addition, it facilitates the elimination of toxins.

The World Health Organization (WHO), The American Academy of Nutrition and Dietetics, The American Cancer Society and several other organizations, have all appealed towards a PBWF eating lifestyle as a suggested healthy habit, in order to decrease the number of million adults' chronic illness worldwide annually. Humans may also consider opting for veggies high protein diet to cure and reverse heart disease, hypertension, and stroke risk factors.

Mass Media marketing introduced to the world's society, the childish habit of labelling a people' groups that use to do, think or prefer same things instead of others, that means if you are thinking of trying for a while a different type of healthy eating, you immediately achieve some funny social stickers.

Vegetarian, Vegan, Pescatarian, Flexitarian... are some example... be careful, we feel all lost without any social label.

It is important to understand that once you decide to take a different approach towards a healthy diet and lifestyle, you will go through times of negative feelings until you proof the benefits of your new healthy journey. As humans, our main aim should be to spread and share as much of our knowledge as possible about a plant-based food culture. We can start by understanding the 2 main categories,

What and which are Macro and Micro Nutrients?

Macros:

Carbs-Fats-Proteins: these are food elements that work together to provide the necessary energy to the human body which support the body to operate and function correctly.

Micro:

Vitamins and Minerals: Vitamins and minerals are essential substances that our bodies need to develop and function normally.

Food care first

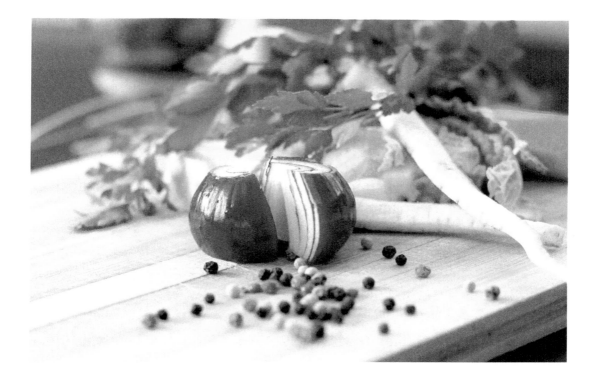

Clean and wash fruit and vegetables properly prior to meal prepping. Do this by soaking you fruit and vegetables in sodium bicarbonate or amuchina and rinse thoroughly. This action helps to disinfect from any pesticides, to prevent foodborne illnesses and to kill any harmful bacteria or parasites. Cooking/Steaming your plant-based food with the benefits of enjoying all the active nutrients in vegetables and delight the full taste of them. A plant-based high protein diet is a suggested healthy alternative to animal-based diets and is the respectful and ethic approach for human, it helps in reducing CO2, decrease animals suffering and last but not least contributes positively towards climate change

Now is the time to focus on which PWBF provide us with the best and highest percentage of proteins:

Beans-Chickpeas high protein content

Seaweed-Algae contain DHA essential fatty acid and protein-

Broccoli vitamins C-K, flavonoids, and protein

Cauliflower high protein, vitamins C-K

Cabbage high protein and vitamins

Brussel sprouts high protein-fiber and vitamins

Spinach leaf high protein, essential amino acids and vitamins

Chia, Hemp, Flax Seeds - High in protein, fiber; omega3 fatty acids source, healthy for skin, hair, help reduce inflammations.

Peanuts - High in protein, peanuts can be roasted, boiled, or baked or as a butter nut.

Wild rice- high in protein and fiber.

Quinoa-Pearled Spelt (pronounced "KEEN-WAH") – a crunchy nutty texture with a mild flavor that is somewhat sweet. A great protein source, which goes great with veg or fruit, in fresh summer salads or hot winter soups.

Tempeh, Tofu and Seitan- have a pleasant rich texture after fermentation or pressing process. They can all be seasoned and are high in protein and fiber.

Veggies' Protein

1) Beans, Legumes and Peas: Beans and legumes are some of the most versatile and nutritious foods you can eat, with more than 25 grams of protein per cup 2) Nuts: Almonds are rich in vitamin E, contain a good amount of calcium, potassium and vitamin B-6, and 10 grams of protein per serving. The most common nuts include almonds, cashews, walnuts, Brazil nuts and pistachios and are a perfect snack when hunger bites.
2) Seeds: A wide range of seeds are extremely nutritious, a single ounce (28 grams) of raw pistachios contains almost 50 percent more protein than one ounce of animal flesh (28 grams), and a serving is also very high in carbohydrates, minerals and go

well with fruit and unsweetened yogurt or vanilla ice cream, for a healthy and tasty breakfast.

3) Berries: Dark chocolate and raspberries have been shown to help prevent heart disease, protect against cancer growth and improve blood flow. A cup of blueberries contains 10 grams of fiber; strawberries contain a remarkable amount of potassium, vitamin K, vitamin C, Thiamine. A half a cup of raspberries contains as much fiber as a cup of cooked spinach.

4) Whole Grains: Whole grains are another optimal plant-based source of protein, especially pearled spelt, buckwheat and quinoa. Pearled spelt contains higher protein content – Buckweat&Quinoa contain all 8 essential aminoacidic our body needs to thrive – Quinoa is gluten free, medium high in protein and a soluble fiber is welcomed for gut health. – all of them have been linked to lower rates of common cancer – and can lower cholesterol levels in the blood.

5) Soy: Soy is a highly nutritious food, containing high amounts of protein, calcium, vitamin C, and many other vitamins and minerals. Some common soy-based foods are tofu (made from processed soybeans), tempeh (made from whole cooked soybeans), and miso soup (made from fermented soybeans).

6) Seaweed: sea vegetables are a kind of algae visible clearly visible in the ocean, highly nutritious and provide many human' health benefits. They can be found on the market in the form of a green powder and a small amount daily should be enough.

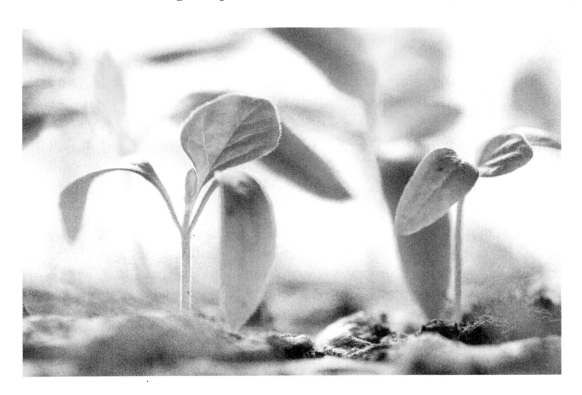

Plant-based & Whole-Food (PBWF)

The term wholefood refers to foods that everyone can eat raw or steamed or boiled (fruit, nuts, seeds, legumes, brown rice, quinoa) as we have seen above. On the other hand, plant-based refers to all green leafy veggies, roots, tubers, radishes, or any other edible plants (onions, sweet potatoes, ginger, beets, garlic, fennel, celery).

Anyone would like to discover the longest-living and healthiest population around the Mother Earth, they will be surprised, that they all have one thing in common: PBWF diet. It goes without saying, that when you find a solution to a vital problem, you first try and understand how the solution is working and then you share your new knowledge and habits with family and friends.

It is important to underline that we are exploring not only a diet, but a completely new lifestyle, made of new healthy habits, new ingredients, new ways to cook and mainly new ways to enjoy life and food.

A good mix between PBWF, steamed, boiled or cooked, represents a perfect meal in terms of right combination of nutrients that humans need to function properly throughout the day.

Meal prep-plans are a matter of culture, traditions, passion, and awareness of undertaking the right steps to improve health, as we unlocked at the beginning of this guide, the no. 1 cause of premature death in America, is in fact, junk food.

It should be a wise behavior, learning how to prepare a healthy and nutrition meal, improving which diet workout plan to choose, watching tutorials, studying and reading to define and achieve our goals... after all the only risk is to get better health, isn't it?

With one simple click it is possible to know how to take care of ourselves better than anyone else, "trying and falling" is the basic pillar of well-living. Set up and start to hear-feel body and mind is not only suggested from several ethical family doctors and nutritionists professionals, but it should be humans' first goal to shut out from boring and unhealthy wheel life.

PBWF eating is one of the best working answers to several questions related to this topic, below you will find practical suggestions on how improve and maintain long term state benefits:

- building a culture of health-wealth
- mindset tips
- list of suggested foods to eat
- organized shopping plan
- storage advice
- meal prep recipes
- 4-week personalized meal plan
- soft workout plan
- powerful allies as I.F.
- cleaning herb' infusion

The best source of proteins are green leaf and whole food, equipped with all the essential amino acids which allow our bodies to heal, build muscle tissue, antibodies, neurotransmitters, enzymes, and much more.

Blaming hormone imbalances for resistant gain weight is unlikely quite common after 30' as American. Cheap fast food, processed and refined food, are the principals responsible, with total absence of daily training and nutritional culture, of this merciless reality. The finale result is to gain toxic body, suffering of fluid retentions and inflammations linked to an excess of toxins, increasing belly and get depressed, dramatic conditions, that is absolutely necessary to reset and reverse.

How to get ride from this body and brain shame?

Strong determination first and powerful awareness to fil knowledge nutrition' gap are the answer.

It may be worth seeking out a professional nutrition course online, or reading a medical guide on this topic, to check out and improve your knowledge of preventive medicine. Any American may find, and this was demonstrated in an AHA analysis, that there is an impressive knowledge gap from family physicians sharing information on nutrition, meaning that patient knowledge on PBWF is virtually absent.

Finding an ethical and professional doctor-nutritionist, becoming more confident with health care and diet are all proof for a healthier future well-being. Knowing that junk food can contain injected hormones, mercury, antibiotics, iron, preservatives...etc...it can be frustrating and unbelievable, but it is unfortunately the reality, the sooner people know about it, the better chance they will have of finding solutions.

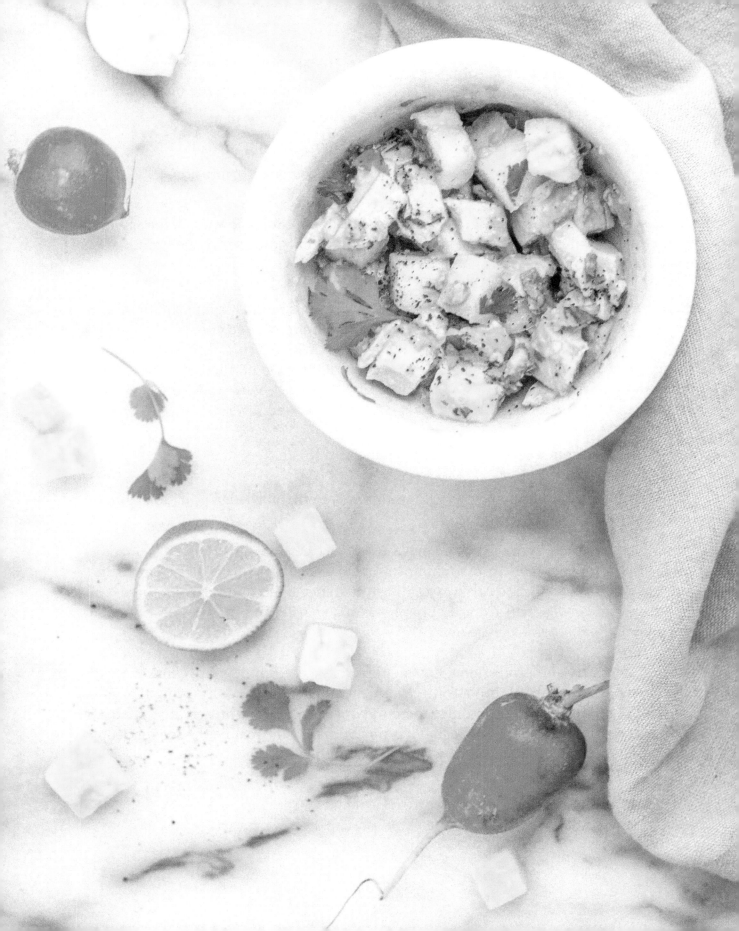

Chapter 2: All About Ph

Measure of the acidity or alkalinity of a fluid is called **pH**, it's the level of hydrogen ion (H+) concentration of standard solution, it can range from 0 to 14, where 0 is most acid, 14 most basic, and 7 is neutral. Human body fluids pH balance, also referred to as acid-alkaline balance, is the level of acids and bases in blood, lungs and kidneys, they play a key role in this process, kidneys help the lungs maintain acid-base balance by excreting acids or bases into the blood, normal blood pH level is between 7 and 7.50. A blood pH imbalance may lead to several health disorder and chronic diseases.

Food' impact on pH

All "food" ingested actually becomes part of the human body, in the blood, in the cells, energy centers, organs, and glands that are responsible for regulating pH levels and general health' state of the persons.

The reason why a PBWF diet is so important in helping to get out of excess weight, and many connected diseases is that it promotes an alkaline environment in our bodies (as opposed to the diet SWE suggests).

Foods that are high in vegetal protein, complex carbohydrates, and fiber help to naturally regulate our pH levels in a way that is more suited for a healthy body.

Following a serious and focused PBWF diet for at least for 12 months, can help to reduce and reverse general indispositions-inflammations, help get back in shape and improve positive mood.

Well balanced pH

A diet with a high acid pH raises the risk of major chronic diseases like, diabetes, osteoporosis, Alzheimer's disease, some cancer and arteriosclerosis. A low acid pH compromises the immune system and weakens the ability to fight bacterial infections.

Consuming too many products containing acid and alkali (alkali-forming substances like soda) can cause a rapid shift in liver function which will cause excessive production of uric acid, an undesirable build-up that is a precursor to arterial disease. It can also cause excessive alkaline ingestion, which can lead to a depletion of acidity in the blood. Too much acid or alkali is not recommended to stay healthy, and it requires that we consume a balanced diet.

Modern lifestyles have led to imbalances in the cells (acidosis) due to the effects of animal-based diet, processed food, ingestion of pesticides, chemical pills, etc. The modern diet is based on excessive consumption of acids (sugar, GMO flour, refined foods, animal products, processed foods, etc.) which deplete the natural alkaline reserves in our blood and body.

Some people will require additional assistance to switch to a more alkaline diet, as they might experience problems with their gastrointestinal system (gut, kidneys, liver) and might need support from professional nutritionist, to carry on this new healthy plan.

The following diet is based on "acid and alkaline-forming foods". Each type of food, when digested and assimilated into the body, produces a different type of energy.

Acid-forming foods include carbonated soft drinks, sugar, GMO flour products, etc. These substances contain acids which, after digested, will increase the acid levels in our blood. Acidic pH causes serious dysfunctions like blood and joint inflammations.

On the other hand, alkaline-forming food is based on fresh fruits, vegetables and whole food. These foods contain enzymes, minerals and vitamins that help to maintain clean and fluid human blood and help with well aging joints.

Lemons can be considered either acid-forming or alkaline-forming depending on the way in which they are consumed. When eaten raw, lemons, will have an alkalizing effect on the body since they are full of enzymes. However, when cooked together with sugar they will create a more acidic result.

The foods listed below are acid-forming and alkaline-forming. They will help to maintain an appropriate pH balance in our bodies.

Acid forming foods: sugar, refined flours, processed foods, alcoholic beverages, red meat, dairy products, (including cured meats like salami, etc.), and soft drinks. Alcohol is very acidic as it contains about 7% alcohol by volume. As a result, it can be considered acid-forming.

Alkaline forming foods: fruits, vegetables, nuts and seeds (including flaxseed), legumes (pulses) wheat germ oil (uncooked), coconut oil/milk/water as well as herbs and spices. Tea and coffee contain alkalizing properties too.

Alkalized body

Human body cells need oxygen to function properly. A body high in alkaline, promotes the healthy life of all its cells, while an acidic body starves its cells of this life-giving component. This means that cells live longer, perform their job as expected and are restored when a large amount of oxygen is available.

Definition of metabolism is the burning of nutrients in the body that would otherwise be stored, with the help of the Oxygen, this burning process also supplies the humans with energy and heat. An alkaline body is more vital, energetic, and warmer. Contrary, an acidic body will be full of stored fats, toxins and definitely colder.

An alkaline environment can drive a more powerful brain, while the brain constitutes about two per cent of human body's weight, it uses 20 per cent of its oxygen and 25 per cent of its energy that is generated by oxygen.

A lack of oxygen is responsible for almost all diseases, bacteria, and fungi flourish in oxygen-starved environments; It has been proved by old research that cancer was caused by a lack of oxygen in cells. Hypertension often occurs when red blood cells are damaged due to low oxygen, which depletes them of the substance that they normally release to relax blood vessels. The human immune system needs a significant amount of oxygen to destroy harmful organisms and flush them from cells.

In an acidic body, calcium does a poor job of developing bone, protein struggles to grow muscle, omega 3 essential fatty acids cannot improve concentration and cognition, iron cannot build red blood cells, there is no part of the body that does not benefit from copious amounts of oxygen. Food nutrients cannot provide your body with any benefits until they are combined with oxygen in our cells.

An alkaline lifestyle is one of the wisest contributions you can make to your health, feeding the human body with an abundance of oxygen should be warmly recommended.

Low pH index

- Lack of minerals & vitamins
- Lack of fatty acids Omega3
- Chemical adding toxins in food, and environment
- Daily stressed routine
- Absence of daily training
- Lack of Sleep and related disorders
- Constipation that leaves toxins accumulating in the colon
- Over the counter & prescription pills, toxins can lead acidic pH

Acidic foods cause a demineralization of the skeleton, and mobilized bone calcium is excreted. This can leave insufficient minerals in the alkaline reserve, main cause of Osteoporosis and several other diseases. Acids pH, cause suffering of several illness and autoimmune diseases as: Systemic lupus, Inflammatory bowel disease, Multiple sclerosis, Arthritis, Psoriasis and Vasculitis.

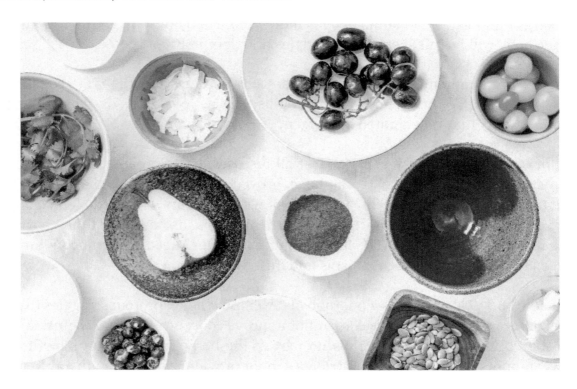

Chapter 3: Shopping Cart

Write down a plant-based & whole-food shopping list, buy enough ingredients, store them in a well-organized pantry and set weekly menus, these are all simple and doable acts. But for many of us, it is the most difficult task to face every week and having an outlined plan is a common "impossible mission".

Here are some pointers for people gathering and matching food in order to sustain new habits and tasty meal prep.

5 Basic Pillars of the Plant-Based Shopping List

1. Eat at least 3 pieces of fruit a day

Seasonal fruit is undoubtedly one of the main sources of healthy nutrients that should not be missing and should always be readily available.

Apples are essential as they go well with all foods. They can be used to prepare green smoothies, porridges, add them to a bowl of cereal and vegetable-based milk, or eat them alone during the day when hunger strikes.

Bananas are allies when it comes to preparing fast, delicious, and healthy smoothies. Remember to choose the ones with brown spots on their skin since they are the best. They are rich in a fundamental mineral called potassium.

Shopping of seasonal fruit and veggies is suggested, so you will ensure sustainability and freshness. In the winter: oranges, kiwi, pomegranates, pineapple, pear and tangerines are preferable.

In summer: Peaches, melons, guava, plums, strawberries, blueberries, watermelons, mango, papaya, grapes, etc. are great in smoothies or juices or shakes mixed with vegetables and nuts for a mouthwatering liquid meal.

Lemons, amazing natural antibiotics, best in the morning with warm water to clean and revitalize the whole body.

Avocados are a slightly salty flavored fruit. They are considered highly for their content of healthy oil and fats, so never leave them out of your shopping cart. They are also quite versatile and can be sued with several recipes.

Ginger is a root to also include in this group, it is anti-inflammatory, and antioxidant. Use it every day in your green infusion, smoothies or meal prep.

2. Buy all kinds of vegetables

Including a large quantity of Plant-Based ingredients in a well-balanced meal prep, is always recommended. It will add more color and taste to any meal.

Below, a list of the most typical and most common Plant-Based foods:

- Green leaves: spinach, arugula,
- Swiss chard, etc.
- Broccoli or cauliflower
- Cabbage
- Zucchini
- Onions
- Garlic
- Aubergines
- Tomatoes
- Cucumber
- Celery
- Artichokes
- Potatoes or potatoes
- Leeks

The idea is to combine raw or cooked vegetables in a rich delicious mixed salad. Season with lemon, extra virgin olive oil, a bit of Himalayan salt and the game is done. A tasty meal with a combination of different textures, colors and flavors.

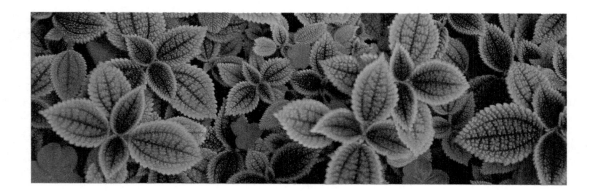

3. Carbohydrates, cereals, grains, and whole meal flour

These nutrients are necessary for the organism' correct function since they provide the necessary energy for our daily life activities. Consuming whole grains is a saluber choice for their high fiber content that provides satiety and lowers its glycemic index. Choose 2 or 3 cereals per week and alternate each day, quinoa, brown rice, amaranth, corn noodles, buckwheat, oats...quinoa vegetable salad is ideal fast, nutritional, and a delicious meal prep. It is recommended that cereal is mixed when consumed since each one provides different nutrients. Remember that it is best to consume them at noon so that you can "burn" them during the day.Within this group, bread is also included. Eat bread made with whole meal flours that will give you more fiber and satiety with a lower glycemic index. You can find several tasty recipes, on the web, for different combinations of gluten-free and whole meal flours.

4. Legumes are the best source of vegetable protein

When eating legumes do the same as with cereals: Choose 2 different ones and consume them alternately during the week. E.g., mix lentils with chickpeas. With lentils, you can prepare hamburgers, include them in salads or make delicious stews. Chickpeas also allow various preparations such as hummus to accompany salads, raw vegetables or as a dip or spread. Use them to make vegan burgers, falafel, include them in salads, or use them in stews. Other legumes that you can consume are green peas, beans, soybeans, and all other beans on the market.

5. Includes nuts and seeds

Although they are last on the list, they are considered an extremely important group for their contribution of proteins, fats, and essential nutrients.

Chia, flax and pumpkin seeds can be used to add to green smoothies, tasty summer salads, hot winter soups and fruit bowls. They are highly antioxidant, anti-inflammatory, and have a high percentage of vitamins and minerals.

Choose nuts such as almonds, walnuts, hazelnuts, cashews (cashews). Being a group of foods with a high protein content make a mix of them and consume a handful every day along with dried fruit, add them to a green smoothie or use them with vegetables to prepare a crispy salad.

Other Foods to Complete Your Plant-Based Shopping List

Preferable 70% dark chocolate, when and if necessary, a shade of sweeter chocolate too.

Coconut oil can be used to spread on gluten-free bread to replace butter.

As for natural sweeteners, use fructose, natural organic honey, or use agave and rice syrups.

Tahini is another food that is used to spread on bread. It is bought ready, or you can make it yourself by processing roasted sesame seeds until their oil begins to spread and they transform into pasta or butter.

Condiments and spices: spices cannot be missing from your pantry. Spices enhance your meals' flavor and boost-heal body and brain functions: ginger, turmeric, curry, mint, rosemary, sage, dill, garlic, onion, paprika. Remember to also add Himalayan salt or another salt that is not refined, to your shopping chart.

Veggie's proteins content

A high protein aliment is when a diet contains a high level of protein content according to one of the following methods:

The percentage of the food that is made up of proteins

The weight percent that is made up of proteins

The number of grams that are produced per 100 grams or milliliters from proteins.

#1: The percentage of the food that is made up of proteins

If a food contains 10% protein on its ingredients list, then only 10% of the total weight or volume in which it's found would be made up from molecules containing proteins. The remaining 90% of the food would be made up of non-protein molecules.

#2: The weight percent that is made up of proteins

If a food contains 12% protein on its ingredients list, then 12% of the total weight or volume in which it's found would be made up from molecules containing proteins. The remaining 88% of the food would be made up of non-protein molecules.

#3: The number of grams that are produced per 100 grams or milliliters from proteins.

This list produces some of the lowest carb fruit options - meaning they have less than five grams of carbs per serving size:

- Avocado 6 g
- Mangoes (2 g)
- Blueberries (5.1 g)
- Raspberries (3.4 g) Grapefruit (3 g)
- Kiwi Fruit (2.8 g)
- Carrots (2 g)
- Pineapples (5.5 g) Limes (2.7 g)
- Watermelon (3.6g)
- Oranges/Orange Juice (0.8 - 1.2 g)
- Nectarine Fruit (3.7 g)
- Cantaloupe (3.8 g)
- Coconut (1.8 g)
- Pink Grapefruit (5.1 g)
- Strawberries (6.3 g)
- Peaches (4.2 g)
- Watermelon Rinds (3.2 g)
- Figs (5.6 g)

Store & Freeze

Nowadays, we are all trying our best to manage healthy habits while controlling expenses, cause by the current pandemic and linked economic stressors. Supporting the immune system through healthy food choices is a good strategy. The human's priority is not just to eat...even several times a day, but to select foods that support our health, which also helps to save money.

A pantry, where replenish cooking and food preparation supplies, can be an extended area of the kitchen and this way our ingredients are easily accessible whenever needed. Flats with large kitchens provide a perfect pantry nook, that is normally tucked away, sheltered and well organized.

Setting up a panty and refrigerator to include more vegetables-based options can help budget & health. The focus should be on plant based, whole foods, such as fresh (or frozen) vegetables and fruit, protein sources that include lentils, peas and beans, whole grains, nuts, and seeds. Long-lasting pantry staples include a variety of beans, chickpeas, pearled spelt, quinoa, and olives. Almond, rice, soy, coconut milks are shelf-stable, and can be great options for many recipes.

Find areas with large open doors and walls that can serve as "tops" that hold several smaller items stacked vertically or horizontally so they are easy and quick to access at your convenience. Shelves can often be used for many different food storages: pea protein powder, spirulina powder, whole grain flours and many others.

Other shelf-stable options include whole-grain pastas, buckwheat noodles, rice, and quinoa. Canned tomatoes, tomato paste, for pasta sauces, hot tasty soups, or veggies prep. Dry spices last a long time, and help to add new flavours to many meals and savour up leftovers to improve taste and further extend your budget. Dedicate a particular pantry section and stock up on budget-friendly frozen vegetables and fruit.

Adding vegetables to meals will make them more digestible and satiating due to the fibre content. Including frozen berries to breakfast cereal or dry-grain mix is cheaper than buying fresh berries. Some frozen fresh vegetable mix options for soups and grain bowls include shredded peas, spinach, potatoes, carrots, beans, and Brussel sprouts.

Buy dried lentils or legumes and fresh veggies and make your own meal…instead of buying canned soup. Lentils are low in saturated fat but high in B9 vitamins, potassium, fiber, antioxidants and proteins. They are also a stately prebiotic for gut microbiome and help to cut down thickset sodium and preservatives of canned soups. Making an important quantity of soup, it's convenient than a single serving, which is why it is suggested to freeze leftovers, this way you have a ready to eat meal prep.

If you're worried about not getting enough protein from vegetables-based diet, it's good to know that 8 ounces (1 cup) of cooked lentils provides about 18 grams of protein, and it has no saturated fat or thickset sodium. Compare that to 4 ounces of minced beef, which provides only 14 grams of protein, no gain fibre, and 11 grams of ill saturated fat.

In the end, vegetables-based diets are famed sources of B9 vitamins, soluble and insoluble fibre, iron, phosphorus, polyunsaturated and monounsaturated fatty acids, veggies options lending themselves to creative cooking: vegetables burgers, stir-fry prep, legumes deeps, stews and soups, peas, corn, and roots salads.

Start looking through the faithful stores and look out for what is on sale that week, and stock it up. It might be a good idea to freeze fresh fruits and vegetables, well cleaned, for later use by storing them properly in the freezer. Don't forget to stock up on sale items such as dried chickpeas, beans, lentils, peas, quinoa and spelt, a budget friendly plant-based diet has many positive effects physical and mentally and can avoid frequent medical checkups.

Plant-based foods	Grams of protein
1 cup cooked/boiled lentils	18
1/2 cup dry red beans	21
1/2 cup chia seeds	18
1/2 cup flax seeds	18
1/2 cup dry black beans	27

Yes or No

Is it a myth that the faithful diet plan has to be acid free?

Yes...almost all human' nutrition should be slightly alkaline, like green and leafy vegetables, including spinach, cabbage, broccoli, peas, asparagus, celery, kale, garlic, onion and potatoes, as well as almost all fruit, nuts, seeds and whole grain.

Remember to drink 8 glasses of water or more per day, so the body can remain hydrated, remove toxins, and leave kidneys enough water to perform their job properly.

Avoid acids like soft drink, soda-based drink, which are full of refined sugar, alcohol, spirits, too much coffee, cow milk, beverages in general should be alkaline or neutral. Fine alkalis are grape, apple, pear, peach, watermelon, mango, in fresh homemade juices or smoothies even adding vegetables and seeds.

Add mineral supplements such as calcium, potassium, and magnesium.

Include whole grain pasta and brown rice, quinoa or pearled spelt, consume daily nuts and seeds to replace junk food. It's suggested that you use pure bitter cacao 70%, herbs or lemon juice, nut butters and pressed olive oil, instead of common unhealthy commercial dressing, as a healthier condiment.

Almond, coconut, rice, or soy milk instead of cow's milk, natural green tea or other herbal infused teas can all be found and are readily available at our local health shops and nowadays even in most supermarkets.

'Eat raw fruits and fresh organic vegetables, well cleaned, as clever fibre' choice.

Drinking pure hot water mixed with lemon and medicinal herbs (thyme, mint, sage, ginger, turmeric) contributes to a sound alkaline detoxed body environment.

A vital point to note is to accept and implement the advices and new habits that can be learned even by following groups on social networks, information that's put into practice, can totally transform, and improve psychophysical health, decrease and reverse the pains of an existing disease or discomfort. Remaining sceptical, stubborn, and refusing to change without trying is like condemning yourself to suffer more and more...it's a behaviour that makes no sense.

The National Library of Medicine, nutritionists guide, popular books, social media groups interview, web channel tutorial...are all available and are a great source of support and help if you are feeling tired an overwhelmed...the only missing attribute is the human willingness to change.

Chapter 4: Health&Food Tips

Pretty goals

Plant-based and whole nutrition is based on vegetables, plants, legumes, whole-grain, nuts, seeds and fruit. By mixing these foods together it is possible to create countless mouthwatering recipes that can motivate and surprise any newbies resulting in a happier diet-journey. Eating plant-based foods helps feeling full for longer and losing weight easier while absorbing only few calories.

This diet-plan is rich in, antioxidants and phytonutrients that are able to protect and better stand human body from chronic diseases like dementia, cardiovascular problems, stroke and joint pain.

It has been shown that the vegetables-based diet burns more calories than other types of diets since it requires less energy for digestion and absorption.

Weight loss: Weight loss is only achievable through a reduction in the intake of bad fats and carbs and starting a serious daily training plan, for these reasons its highly recommended to follow a plant-based diet plan.

More strength: A high protein plant-based diet helps you gain more muscle mass, making you bulkier and more athletic. If you are afraid to switch to green foods because for some reason or other you cannot live without animal products such as eggs and milk, remember that all plants offer the same benefits as animal products. In addition, a plant-based diet allows you to absorb nutrients better since you're cutting out the unhealthy fats and refined sugars from your diet.

Cardiovascular diseases: High protein diets are beneficial for healthy heart function and cardiovascular system because they help your heart gain new muscle mass while regulating blood pressure levels. Also, higher protein vegetables-based intake lowers the levels of triglycerides in your blood which makes you less susceptible to cardiovascular illness.

Dementia: Dementia is one of the most common diseases worldwide. In a study conducted by a group of vegans, it was revealed that they had lower rates of dementia than non-vegan participants. Psychiatric patients processed foods containing animal products more slowly and logically than those who are vegetarian or vegan.

Stroke: Many studies have revealed that a high protein diet raises your risk of stroke. Strokes are caused by a blockage in blood vessels, and high protein diets can cause hardening of the arteries which leads to clots forming in the blood, moving towards the heart or brain. Also, you must be aware that some proteins like eggs or milk contain cholesterol which can raise your risk of stroke as well.

Cancer: Decrease the cancer risk, because plant-based diet is full of phytonutrients and antioxidants, also warmly recommended by many American health associations to prevent and stop the rise of several cancers.

Immune system boost

Many doctors and health experts have accepted that plant-based diet can play an important role in how well your body functions. It is not necessarily true that if you eat a healthy diet then your immune system will be at its strongest possible state. On the contrary, some evidence suggests that unhealthy diets are associated with weaker immune systems.

One of the most known causes for this is due to high levels of saturated fat in a diet, which has been shown to decrease the function of white blood cells and cause inflammation as well as other disease-causing effects in the long term.

Plant-based diets are known to suppress the production of inflammatory compounds in the body, as well as being low in saturated fat content and high in essential nutrients, including omega-3 fatty acids. This means that if you eat a healthy diet that includes a whole range of plant foods, then your immune system will remain strong and healthy.

Top recovery

1. Drink a juice or smoothie with high content of protein, fiber and light carbs after each workout.
2. Eat healthy foods within one hour of working out to start replenishing glycogen stores and fuel your muscles.
3. Replace lost fluids with water or coconut water to stay hydrated - aim for 16 ounces per pound lost or just over two liters on average per day for the next few days.
4. Keep an eye on calories by eating enough but not too much - 2,000 calories are a good starting point for the next few days if you're trying to gain weight or 1,800 if you're trying to lose weight).
5. Eat protein with each meal to help repair muscles.
6. Stretch to avoid sore muscles and prevent injury or stiffness in muscles and joints.
7. Sleep a full night, as resting allows the body to repair itself from the workout
8. Use the day after a workout as an active recovery by taking a walk or doing yoga or light stretching
9. Alter your workout routine so you don't overtrain your body (fast-twitch muscle fibers recover from a heavy lifting session much faster than slow-twitch).
10. Listen to your body - If it feels like you've pushed yourself too hard, take a rest day or adjust your workout routine

Exercise Poses

1. The cat stretch

Your spine responds best to stretching when you don't bounce right away. That's why we commended starting off with a stretch like this one, which needs to be held for fifteen seconds at a time before bouncing up and down.

2. The low back stretch

For even better lower back flexibility, focus on the lumbar spine instead of the thoracic spine by performing this stretch starting with your hand on the floor (you can also start from hands on knees).

3. The forward bend stretch

This one is for the more advanced since it requires a certain level of flexibility already at your fingertips. It's also tough for many people to hold the stretch for more than 30 seconds at first. So, either shorten the time you're holding the stretch or work up to it gradually and build up your strength in small increments.

4. The lumbar roll

We know that rolling your lower back is not one of those things everybody likes to do but trust us on this one: doing this will make you feel awesome! Just lay on your back and wiggle those around a little bit, taking care not to roll into a proper backbend but instead keep that natural curve in your lower back. (Try this with an elbow wedge under your shoulder blades.)

5. The bridge twist

This one is also an advanced skill since it requires not only flexibility in your lower back but also a certain degree of strength. Try this one while holding yourself up with your arms, which is much easier than using just your legs.

6. The cat-camel exercise

This is a more dynamic stretch than the others on the list so far and should be done for 30 seconds at a time instead of fifteen seconds (otherwise you risk doing more harm than good). The key here is to slowly tense and release different parts of your body without bouncing around too much – nice and controlled! This gives you a perfect base for all those lower back stretches above.

7. The pigeon pose

This one is very similar to the cat-camel stretch, but with a few key differences: instead of slowly releasing all tension, you're slowly starting to build up that tension inside of your lower back. This will make this stretch even more effective than the others described first.

8. The hamstring stretch

If you're struggling with tight hamstrings, try out this stretch (which should also be held for thirty seconds at a time). Resting your knee on something like a pillow will allow your back to relax and loosen up without straining you too much. Like with many other stretches here as well: start off slow and gradually build it up!

9. The downward dog pose

This is a similar stretch as the pigeon, but more advanced than the ones on this list so far. This means that you should probably start with the pigeon or other easier exercises before trying this one out.

10. The seagull balance

If you're feeling extra flexible, you can do something like this pose, which combines many of the stretches already described into one ultra-effective exercise! You can increase flexibility in your lower back even further by doing this with your feet off the ground and using only an edge to keep yourself balanced (like a doorway or armrest).

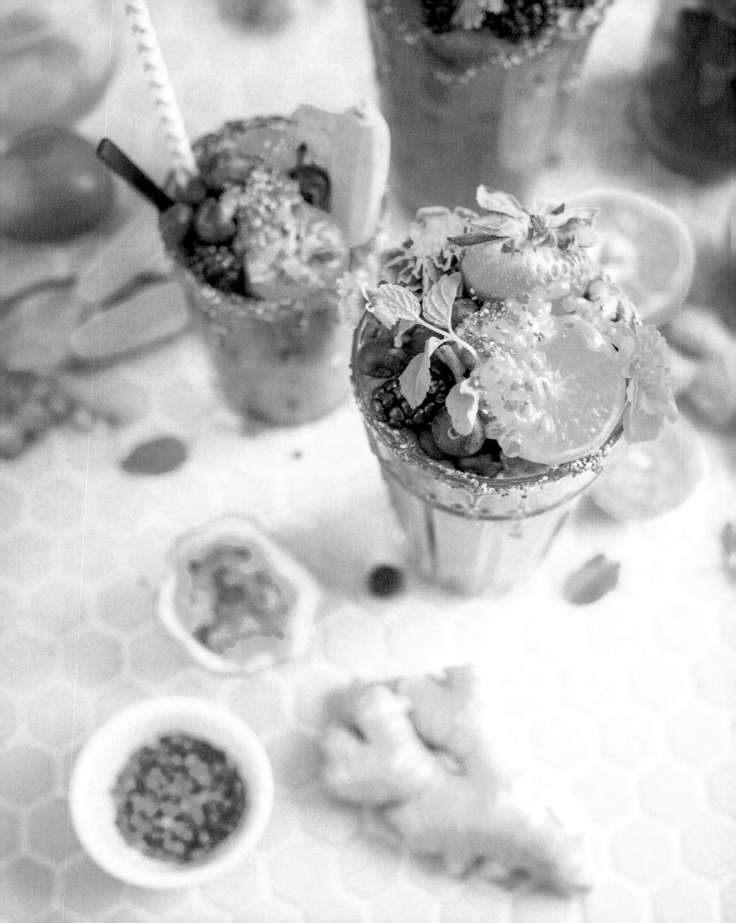

Chapter 5: Breakfast, Smoothies, Juices And Shakes

1. Quinoa Black Beans Breakfast Bowl

Preparation Time: 15 Minutes

Cooking Time: 25 Minutes

Servings: 1

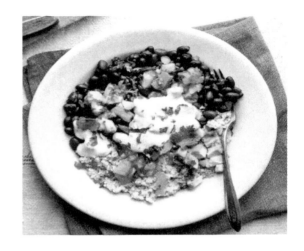

Ingredients:

- 1/4 cup brown quinoa, rinsed well
- Salt to taste
- 1 tbsp plant-based yogurt
- ½ lime, juiced
- 1 tbsp chopped fresh cilantro
- 1 (5 oz) can black beans, drained and rinsed 1 tbsp tomato salsa
- ¼ small avocado, pitted, peeled, and sliced 1 radish, shredded
- 1/4 tbsp pepitas (pumpkin seeds)

Directions:

1. Cook the quinoa with 2 cups of slightly salted water in a medium pot over medium heat or until the liquid absorbs, 15 minutes.
2. Spoon the quinoa into serving bowls and fluff with a fork.
3. In a small bowl, mix the yogurt, lime juice, cilantro, and salt. Divide this mixture on the quinoa and top with beans, salsa, avocado, radishes, and pepitas.
4. Serve immediately.

Nutrition:

Calories: 131   Fats: 3.5g   Carbs: 20g   Proteins: 6.5g

2. Corn Griddle Cakes with Tofu Mayonnaise

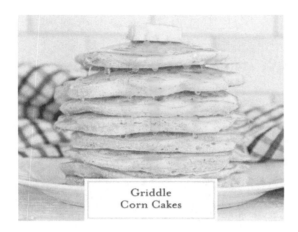
Griddle
Corn Cakes

Preparation Time: 15 Minutes

Cooking Time: 35 Minutes

Servings: 1

Ingredients:

- 1 tbsp flax seed powder + 3 tbsp water
- 1 cup water or as needed
- 1 cup yellow cornmeal
- 1 tsp salt
- 1 tsp baking powder
- 1 tbsp olive oil for frying
- 1 cup tofu mayonnaise for serving

Directions:

1. In a medium bowl, mix the flax seed powder with water and allow thickening
2. for 5 minutes to form the flax egg.
3. Mix in the water and then whisk in the cornmeal, salt, and baking powder until soup texture forms but not watery.
4. Heat a quarter of the olive oil in a griddle pan and pour in a quarter of the batter. Cook until set and golden brown beneath, 3 minutes. Flip the cake and cook the other side until set and golden brown too.
5. Plate the cake and make three more with the remaining oil and batter.
6. Top the cakes with some tofu mayonnaise before serving.

Nutrition:

Calories: 896   Fats 50.7g   Carbs: 91.6g   Proteins: 17.3g

3. Savory Breakfast Salad

Preparation Time: 15 to 30 Minutes

Cooking Time: 20 Minutes

Servings: 1

Ingredients:

- For the sweet potatoes:
- Sweet potato: 2 smalls
- Salt and pepper: 1 pinch
- Coconut oil: 1 tbsp
- For the Dressing:
- Lemon juice: 3 tbsp
- Salt and pepper: 1 pinch each
- Extra virgin olive oil: 1 tbsp
- For the Salad: Mixed greens: 4 cups
- For Serving s: Hummus: 4 tbsp Blueberries: 1 cup
- Ripe avocado: 1 medium
- Fresh chopped parsley
- Hemp seeds: 2 tbsp

Directions:

1. Take a large skillet and apply gentle heat
2. Add sweet potatoes, coat them with salt and pepper and pour some oil Cook till sweet potatoes turns browns
3. Take a bowl and mix lemon juice, salt, and pepper Add salad, sweet potatoes, and the serving together Mix well, dress and serve

Nutrition:

Calories: 523   Carbs: 57.6g   Proteins: 7.5g   Fats: 37.6g

4. Almond Plum Oats Overnight

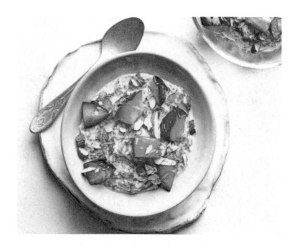

Preparation Time: 15 to 30 Minutes

Cooking Time: 10 Minutes

Servings: 1

Ingredients:

- Rolled oats: 60g
- Plums: 3 ripe and chopped
- Almond milk: 300ml
- Chia seeds: 1 tbsp
- Nutmeg: a pinch
- Vanilla extract: a few drops
- Whole almonds: 1 tbsp roughly chopped

Directions:

1. Add oats, nutmeg, vanilla extract, almond milk, and chia seeds to a bowl and mix well
2. Add in cubed plums and cover and place in the fridge for a night Mix the oats well next morning and add into the serving bowl.
3. Serve with your favorite toppings.

Nutrition:

Calories: 248   Carbs: 24.7g   Proteins: 9.5g   Fats: 10.8g

5. High Protein Toast

Preparation Time: 30 Minutes

Cooking Time: 15 Minutes

Servings: 1

Ingredients:
- White bean: 1 drained and rinsed
- Cashew cream: ½ cup
- Miso paste: 1 ½ tbsp
- Toasted sesame oil: 1 tsp
- Sesame seeds: 1 tbsp
- Spring onion: 1 finely sliced
- Lemon: 1 half for the juice and half wedged to serve Rye bread: 4 slices toasted

Directions:
1. In a bowl add sesame oil, white beans, miso, cashew cream, and lemon juice and mash using a potato masher.
2. Make a spread.
3. Spread it on a toast and top with spring onions and sesame seeds Serve with lemon wedges.

Nutrition:

Calories: 332   Carbs: 44.5g   Proteins: 14.5g   Fats: 9.25g

6. Hummus Carrot Sandwich

Preparation Time: 30 Minutes

Cooking Time: 25 Minutes

Servings: 1

Ingredients:

- Chickpeas: 1 cup can drain and rinsed
- Tomato: 1 small sliced
- Cucumber: 1 sliced
- Avocado: 1 sliced
- Cumin: 1 tsp
- Carrot: 1 cup diced
- Maple syrup: 1 tsp
- Tahini: 3 tbsp
- Garlic: 1 clove
- Lemon: 2 tbsp
- Extra-virgin olive oil: 2 tbsp
- Salt: as per your need
- Bread slices: 4

Directions:

1. Add carrot to the boiling hot water and boil for 15 minutes Blend boiled carrots, maple syrup, cumin, chickpeas, tahini, olive oil, salt, and garlic together in a blender.
2. Add in lemon juice and mix.
3. Add to the serving bowl and you can refrigerate for up to 5 days In between two bread slices, spread hummus and place 2-3 slices of cucumber, avocado, and tomato and serve.

Nutrition:

Calories: 490   Carbs: 53.15g   Proteins: 14.1g   Fats: 27.g

7. <Overnight Oats

Preparation Time: 30 Minutes
Cooking Time: 15 Minutes
Servings: 1

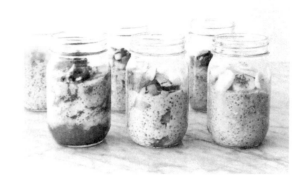

Ingredients:

- Cinnamon: a pinch
- Almond milk: 200ml
- Porridge oats: 120g
- Maple syrup: 1 tbsp
- Pumpkin seeds 1 tbsp
- Chia seeds: 1 tbsp

Directions:

1. Add all the ingredients to the bowl and combine well Cover the bowl and place it in the fridge overnight Pour more milk in the morning. Serve with your favorite toppings

Nutrition:

Calories: 298   Carbs: 32.3g   Proteins: 10.2g   Fats: 12.7g

8. Avocado Miso Chickpeas Toast

Preparation Time: 30 Minutes

Cooking Time: 15 Minutes

Servings: 1

Ingredients:

- Chickpeas: 400g drained and rinsed
- Avocado: 1 medium
- Toasted sesame oil: 1 tsp
- White miso paste: 1 ½ tbsp
- Sesame seeds: 1 tbsp
- Spring onion: 1 finely sliced
- Lemon: 1 half for the juice and half wedged to serve Rye bread: 4 slices toasted

Directions:

1. In a bowl add sesame oil, chickpeas, miso, and lemon juice and mash using a potato masher.
2. Roughly crushed avocado in another bowl using a fork Add the avocado to the chickpeas and make a spread it on a toast and top with spring onion and sesame seeds Serve with lemon wedges.

Nutrition:

Calories: 456   Carbs: 33.3 g   Proteins: 14.6 g   Fats: 26.6 g

9. Banana Malt Bread

1. **Preparation Time**: 30 Mins
2. **Cooking Time**: 1 H 20 Mins
3. **Servings**: 1

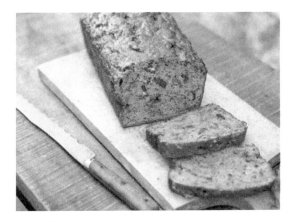

Ingredients:

- Hot strong black tea: 120ml
- Malt extract: 150g plus extra for brushing
- Bananas: 2 ripe mashed
- Sultanas: 100g
- Pitted dates: 120g chopped
- Plain flour: 250g
- Soft dark brown sugar: 50g
- Baking powder: 2 tsp

Directions:

1. Preheat the oven to 140C
2. Line the loaf tin with the baking paper
3. Brew tea and include sultanas and dates to it Take a small pan and heat the malt extract and gradually add sugar to it Stir continuously and let it cook
4. In a bowl, add flour, salt, and baking powder and now top with sugar extract, fruits, bananas, and tea
5. Mix the batter well and add to the loaf tin
6. Bake the mixture for an hour
7. Brush the bread with extra malt extract and let it cool down before removing from the tin
8. When done, wrap in a foil; it can be consumed for a week

Nutrition:

Calories: 194   Carbs: 43.3 g   Proteins: 3.4 g   Fats: 0.3 g

10. Banana Vegan Bread

Preparation Time: 30 Minutes

Cooking Time: 1 Hour and 15 Minutes

Servings: 1

Ingredients:

- Overripe banana:
- 3 large mashed
- All-purpose flour: 200 g
- Unsweetened non-dairy milk: 50 ml
- White vinegar: ½ tsp
- Ground flaxseed: 10 g
- Ground cinnamon: ¼ tsp
- Granulated sugar: 140 g
- Vanilla: ¼ tsp
- Baking powder: ¼ tsp
- Baking soda: ¼ tsp
- Salt: ¼ tsp
- Canola oil: 3 tbsp
- Chopped walnuts: ½ cup

Directions:

1. Preheat the oven to 350F and line the loaf pan with parchment paper Mash bananas using a fork
2. Take a large bowl, and add in mash bananas, canola oil, oat milk, sugar, vinegar, vanilla, and ground flax seed
3. Also whisk in baking powder, cinnamon, flour, and salt Add batter to the loaf pan and bake for 50 minutes Remove from pan and let it sit for 10 minutes Slice when completely cooled down.

Nutrition:

Calories: 240   Carbs: 40.3g   Proteins: 2.8g   Fats: 8.2g

11.   Fruity Smoothie

Preparation Time: 10 Minutes

Cooking time: 0 minute

Servings: 1

Ingredients:
- ¾ cup soy yogurt
- ½ cup pineapple juice
- 1 cup pineapple chunks
- 1 cup raspberries, sliced
- 1 cup blueberries, sliced

Direction:
1. Process the ingredients in a blender.
2. Chill before serving.

Nutrition:

Calories 279	Cholesterol 4 mg	Dietary	Sugars 46 g
Fat 2 g	Sodium 149 mg	Fiber 7 g	Potassium 719 mg
Saturated Fat 0 g	Carbohydrate 56 g	Protein 12 g	

12. Protein Hot Chocolate

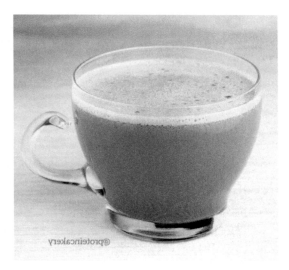

Preparation time: 2 minutes

Cooking time: 2 minutes

Servings: 1

Ingredients:

- 1 scoop chocolate whey protein powder
- 1 cup unsweetened vanilla almond milk
- 3/4 cup water
- 1 tsp unsweet cocoa powder

Directions:

1. Combine all ingredients in a small sauce pot and pout on medium heat.
2. Stir consistently while mixture heats thoroughly, about 3 minutes.
3. Scoop out a tiny portion to taste and test heat. Remove from heat and pour into mug. Sip and enjoy.

Nutrition:

Calories: 145   Fat: 3 g   Carbohydrates: 6 g   Protein: 24 g

13. Iced Vanilla Chai Tea

Preparation time: 3minutes

Cooking time: 0 minutes

Total Time: 3 minutes

Servings: 1

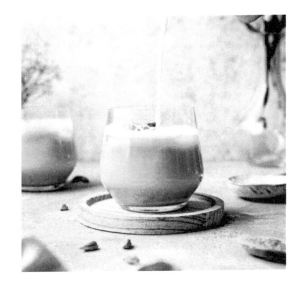

Ingredients:

- bag decaf chai tea
- scoop vanilla whey protein powder
- cup water
- 1/2 cup ice
- 1-3 tsp sweetener

Directions:

1. Steep tea in water for 4 minutes per package Directions. Set aside to let cool to room temperature.
2. Pour tea in a shaker cup with vanilla protein powder and shake well. Pour over ice. Taste and add sweetener if desired.

Nutrition:

Calories: 110   Fat: 1 g   Carbohydrates: 5 g   Protein: 25 g

14. Friendly Creamy Hot Cocoa

Preparation time: 5 minutes

Cooking time: 0 minutes

Servings: 1

Ingredients:
- 1/4 cup low-fat cottage cheese
- scoop whey vanilla protein powder
- 1/2 tsp caramel extract
- 1/2 tsp almond extract
- cup water
- 6 ice cubes

Directions:
1. Combine all ingredients in a blender and blend on high until smooth.

Nutrition:

Calories: 145   Fat: 1 g   Carbohydrates: 6 g   Protein: 29 g

15. Chocolate Milk

Preparation time: 5 minutes
Cooking time: 0 minutes
Servings: 4

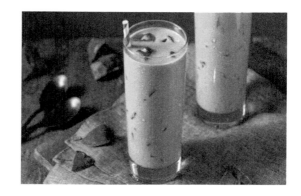

Ingredients:

- 4 cups unsweetened chocolate almond milk
- 4 scoops chocolate protein powder
- 2 tablespoons cocoa powder
- 1 cup ice (optional)

Directions:

1. In a blender, combine the almond milk, protein powder, and cocoa powder and blend until smooth.
2. Serve over ice (if using) or blend the ice into the milk mixture until it achieves your desired consistency.

Nutrition:

calories: 171   fat: 4.0g   protein: 27.0g   carbs: 9.0g net

carbs: 7.0g   fiber: 2.0g

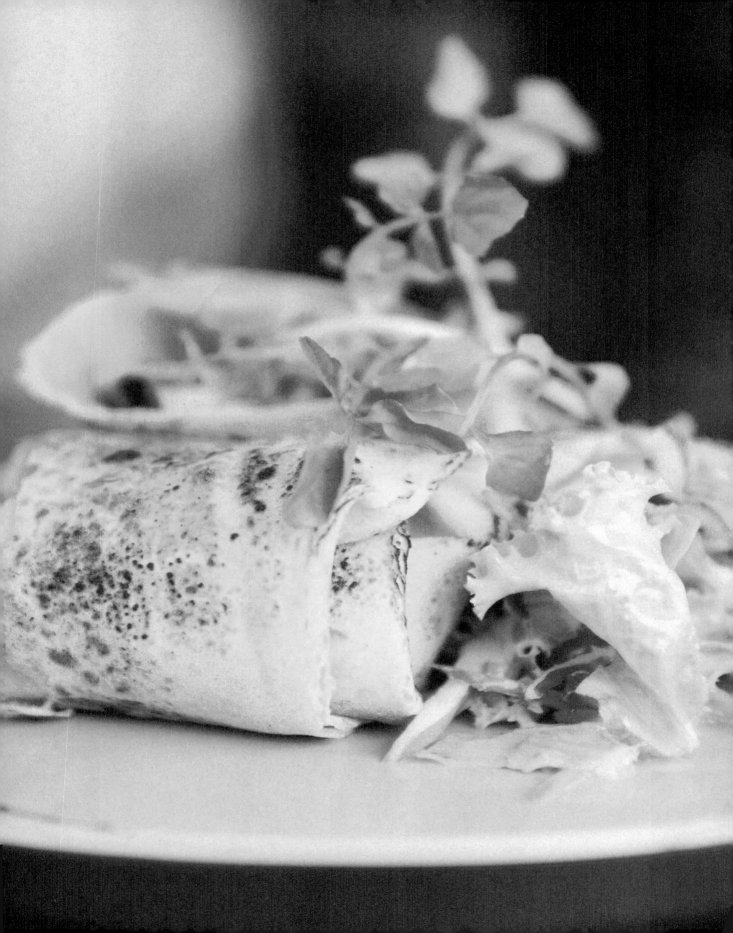

Chapter 6: Snacks and Sides

16.   Mango and Banana Shake

Preparation time: 10 mins

Cooking time: 0 mins

Servings: 2

Ingredients:
- 1 Banana, Sliced and Frozen
- 1 Cup Frozen Mango Chunks
- 1 Cup Almond Milk
- 1 Tbsp. Maple Syrup
- 1 Tsp Lime Juice
- 2-4 Raspberries for Topping
- Mango Slice for Topping

Directions
1. In blender, pulse banana, mango with milk, maple syrup, lime juice until
2. smooth but still thick
3. Add more liquid if needed.
4. Pour shake into 2 bowls.
5. Top with berries and mango slice.
6. Enjoy!

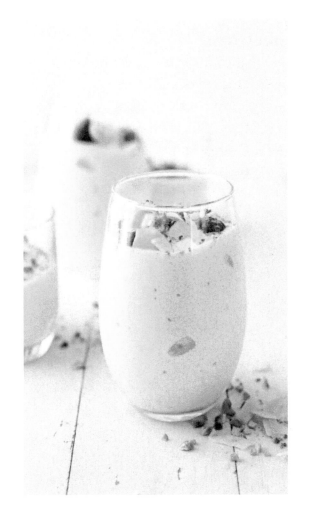

Nutrition:

Protein: 5% 8 kcal   Fat: 11% 18 kcal   Carbohydrates: 85% 140 kcal

17. Avocado Toast with Flaxseeds

Preparation time: 5 mins.

Servings: 3

Cooking time: 0 mins

Ingredients:

- 3 slice of whole grain bread
- 1 large avocado, ripe
- ¼ cup chopped parsley
- 1 tbsp. flax seeds
- 1 tbsp. sesame seeds
- 1 tbsp. lime juice

Directions:

1. First, toast your piece of bread.
2. Remove the avocado seed.
3. Slice half avocado and mash half avocado with fork in bowl.
4. Spread mashed avocado on 2 toasted breads.
5. Place avocado slice on 1 toast.
6. Top with flax seeds and sesame seeds.
7. Drizzle lime juice and chopped parsley on top.
8. Serve and enjoy!

Nutrition:

Protein: 12% 31 kcal   Fat: 49% 124 kcal   Carbohydrates: 39% 98kcal

18. Avocado Hummus

Preparation time: 10 mins

Servings: 4

Cooking time: 0 mins

Ingredients

- 2 Ripe Avocados
- ½ Cup Coconut Cream
- ¼ Cup Sesame Paste
- ½ Lemon Juice
- 1 Tsp. Clove, Pressed
- ½ Tsp Ground Cumin
- ½ Tsp Salt
- ¼ Tsp Ground Black Pepper

Directions

1. Cut the avocado lengthways and remove seed from the fruit.
2. Put all ingredients in a blender or food processor and mix until thoroughly smooth.
3. Add more cream, lemon juice or water if you want to have a looser texture.
4. Adjust seasonings as needed.
5. Serve with naan and enjoy.

Nutrition:

Protein: 6% 21 kcal   Carbohydrates: 16% 57 kcal   Fat: 79% 289 kcal

19. Plant Based Crispy Falafel

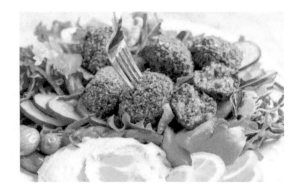

Preparation time: 20 mins

Cooking time: 30 mins

Servings: 8

Ingredients

- 1 tbsp. extra-virgin olive oil
- 1 cup dried chickpeas soaked for 24 hours in the refrigerator 1 cup cauliflower, chopped
- ½ cup red onion, chopped
- ½ cup packed fresh parsley
- 2 cloves garlic, quartered
- 1 tsp. sea salt
- ½ tsp. ground black pepper
- ½ tsp. ground cumin
- ¼ tsp. ground cinnamon

Directions

1. Preheat oven to 375° F.
2. In a food processor, mix chickpeas, cauliflower, onion, parsley, garlic, salt, pepper, cumin seeds, cinnamon, and olive oil until mixture is smooth.
3. Take 2 tbsps. of mixture and make the falafel into small patties.
4. Keep falafel on greased baking tray.
5. Bake falafel for about 25 to 30 minutes in preheated oven until golden brown from both sides.
6. Once cooked remove from oven.
7. Serve hot fresh vegetable salad and enjoy!

Nutrition:

Protein: 16% 19 kcal   Fat: 24% 29 kcal   Carbohydrates: 60% 71kcal

20. Waffles with Almond Flour

Preparation time: 15 mins

Servings: 4

Cooking time: 15 mins

Ingredients

- 1 cup almond milk
- 2 tbsps. chia seeds
- 2 tsp lemon juice
- 4 tbsps. coconut oil
- 1/2 cup almond flour
- 2 tbsps. maple syrup
- Cooking spray or cooking oil

Directions

1. Mix coconut milk with lemon juice in a mixing bowl.
2. Leave it for 5-8 minutes on room temperature to turn it into butter milk.
3. Once coconut milk is turned into butter milk, add chai seeds into milk and whisk together.
4. Add other ingredients in milk mixture and mix well.
5. Preheat a waffle iron and spray it with coconut oil spray.
6. Pour 2 tbsp. of waffle mixture into the waffle machine and cook until golden.
7. Top with some berries and serve hot.
8. Enjoy with black coffee!

Nutrition:

Protein: 5% 15 kcal   Carbohydrates: 23% 66kcal   Fat: 71% 199 kcal

CHAPTER 6

21.   Mint and Avocado Smoothie

Preparation time: 10 mins

Servings: 2

Cooking time: 0 minutes

Ingredients

- 1 cup coconut water
- 1/2 lemon juice
- ½ cup cucumber
- 1 cup mint. fresh
- 1/2 medium size avocado
- I/2 tsp maple syrup
- 1 cup ice

Directions

1. Place all ingredients into a blender, cover lid and blend until smooth.
2. Blend on high speed until smoothie has fluffy texture.
3. Pour smoothie in glass and top with mint leaves.
4. Serve and enjoy!

Nutrition:

Protein: 6% 7 kcal   Carbohydrates: 44% 55 kcal   Fat: 51% 64 kcal

22. Simple Banana Fritters

Preparation time: 15 mins

Cooking time: 20 mins

Servings: 8

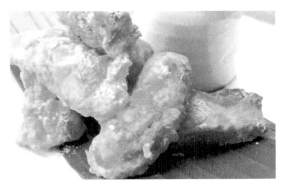

Ingredients

- 4 Bananas
- 3 Tbsps. Maple Syrup
- ¼ Tsp. Cinnamon Powder
- ¼ Tsp. Nutmeg
- 1 Cup Coconut Flour

Directions

1. Preheat oven to 350° F.
2. Mash the bananas in a large mixing bowl along with maple syrup, cinnamon, nutmeg powder and coconut flour.
3. Mix all the ingredients well.
4. Take 2 tbsps. mixture and make small 1-inch-thick fritters from this mixture.
5. Place fritters in greased baking tray.
6. Bake fritters in preheated oven for about 10-15 minutes until golden from both sides.
7. Once done, take them out of the oven.
8. Serve with coconut cream.
9. Enjoy!

Nutrition:

Protein: 3% 3 kcal

Carbohydrates: 69% 75 kcal

Fat: 28% 30 kcal

23.   Coconut and Blueberries Ice Cream

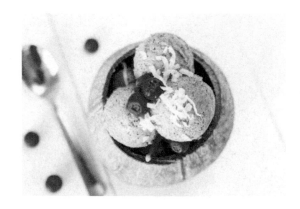

Preparation time: 5 mins

Cooking time: 0 mins

Servings: 4

Ingredients

- 1/4 Cup Coconut Cream
- 1 Tbsp. Maple Syrup
- ¼ Cup Coconut Flour
- 1 Cup Blueberries
- ¼ Cup Blueberries for Topping

Directions

1. Put ingredients into food processor and mix well on high speed.
2. Pour mixture in silicon molds and freeze in freezer for about 2-4 hours.
3. Once balls are set remove from freezer.
4. Top with berries.
5. Serve cold and enjoy!

Nutrition:

Protein: 3% 4 kcal   Carbohydrates: 57% 86 kcal   Fat: 40% 60 kcal

24. Avocado Chaat

Preparation Time: 15 Minutes

Serving: 4

Cooking Time: 5 Minutes

Ingredients:

- 4 Avocado, peeled and diced into bite-sized chunks 2 tsp. Chaat masala
- 1 Lime, juiced
- ½ tsp sea salt
- Coconut yogurt to serve

Directions:

1. 1 Place all together the ingredients in a large bowl and shake them well
2. Now serve it with some coconut yogurt if you desire

Nutrition:

Calories: 234   Fat: 21g   Protein: 3g   Carbohydrates: 12g

25. Crispy Brinjal "Bacon"

Preparation Time: 15 Minutes

Servings: 4

Cooking Time: 40 Minutes

Ingredients:

- 1 medium Eggplant
- 1 ½ tbsp. Tamari
- 1 tbsp. Vegan Worcestershire
- 1 tsp. Smoked paprika
- 1 pinch Garlic powder
- 1 tbsp. Maple syrup
- 2 tbsp. Avocado oil
- 2 tsp. Liquid smoke
- 1 pinch Sea salt
- ½ tsp. Black pepper, freshly cracked

Directions:

1. Take an eggplant and sliced it in half
2. Chop down the eggplant in small size
3. Prepare the sauce by adding the ingredient Worcestershire sauce, maple syrup, paprika, garlic powder, sea salt, black pepper into a bowl
4. Place the sauce onto the eggplant and sprinkle black pepper 5. Cook till the eggplant looks crispy and red 6. For more crisps, let it cool down after you put away heat

Nutrition:

Calories: 28   Fat: 2g   Carbohydrates: 2g   Protein: 0.3g

26. Pomegranate Flower Sprouts

Preparation Time: 15 Minutes
Cooking Time: 15 Minutes
Servings: 2

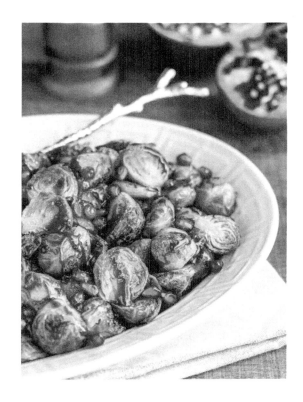

Ingredients:
- 3 tbsp. Pomegranate molasses
- 150 g Flower sprouts
- Vegetable oil for deep-frying
- A pinch Sea salt flakes
- A pinch Pul Biber

Directions:
1. Warm the oil in the pan and when enough heat, add flower sprouts
2. Just fry them for 30 seconds
3. Add them into the bowl with other ingredients and mix 4. Serve right away

Nutrition:

Calories: 202   Fat: 11g   Carbohydrates: 19g   Protein: 3g

27. Banana Curry

Preparation Time: 15 Minutes

Servings: 3

Cooking Time: 15 Minutes

Ingredients:
- 2 tablespoons olive oil
- 2 yellow onions, chopped
- 8 garlic cloves, minced
- 2 tablespoons curry powder
- 1 tablespoon ground ginger
- 1 tablespoon ground cumin
- 1 teaspoon ground turmeric
- 1 teaspoon ground cinnamon
- 1 teaspoon red chili powder
- Salt and ground black pepper, to taste
- 2/3 cup soy yogurt
- 1 cup tomato puree
- 2 bananas, peeled and sliced
- 3 tomatoes, chopped finely
- ¼ cup unsweetened coconut flakes

Directions:
1. In a large pan, heat the oil over medium heat and sauté onion for about 4–5 minutes.
2. Add the garlic, curry powder, and spices, and sauté for about 1minute.
3. Add the soy yogurt and tomato sauce and bring to a gentle boil.
4. Stir in the bananas and simmer for about 3 minutes.
5. Stir in the tomatoes and simmer for about 1–2 minutes.
6. Stir in the coconut flakes and immediately remove from the heat.
7. Serve hot.

Nutrition:

Calories: 382   Fat: 18g   Carbohydrates: 53g   Protein: 9g

28. Mushroom Curry

Preparation Time: 15 Minutes

Servings: 3

Cooking Time: 20 Minutes

Ingredients:

- 2 cups tomatoes, chopped
- 1 green chili, chopped
- 1 teaspoon fresh ginger, chopped
- ¼ cup cashews
- 2 tablespoons canola oil
- ½ teaspoon cumin seeds
- ¼ teaspoon ground coriander
- ¼ teaspoon ground turmeric
- ¼ teaspoon red chili powder
- 1½ cups fresh shiitake mushrooms, sliced
- 1½ cups fresh button mushrooms, sliced
- 1 cup frozen corn kernels
- 1¼ cups water
- ¼ cup unsweetened coconut milk
- Salt and ground black pepper, to taste

Directions:

1. In a food processor, add the tomatoes, green chili, ginger, and cashews, and pulse until a smooth paste form.
2. In a pan, heat the oil over medium heat and sauté the cumin seeds for about 1 minute.
3. Add the spices and sauté for about 1 minute.
4. Add the tomato paste and cook for about 5 minutes.
5. Stir in the mushrooms, corn, water, and coconut milk, and bring to a boil.
6. Cook for about 10–12 minutes, stirring occasionally.
7. Season with salt and black pepper and remove from the heat.
8. Serve hot.

Nutrition:

Calories: 311   Fat: 20g   Carbohydrates: 32g   Protein: 8g

29. Veggie Combo

Preparation Time: 15 Minutes

Servings: 4

Cooking Time: 25 Minutes

Ingredients:
- 1 tablespoon olive oil
- 1 small yellow onion, chopped
- 1 teaspoon fresh thyme, chopped
- 1 garlic clove, minced
- 8 ounces fresh button mushroom, sliced
- 1 pound Brussels sprouts
- 3 cups fresh spinach
- 4 tablespoons walnuts
- Salt and ground black pepper, to taste

Directions:
1. In a large skillet, heat the oil over medium heat and sauté the onion for about 3–4 minutes.
2. Add the thyme and garlic and sauté for about 1 minute.
3. Add the mushrooms and cook for about 15 minutes, or until caramelized.
4. Add the Brussels sprouts and cook for about 2–3 minutes.
5. Stir in the spinach and cook for about 3–4 minutes.
6. Stir in the walnuts, salt, and black pepper, and remove from the heat.
7. Serve hot.

Nutrition:

Calories: 153   Protein: 8g   Carbohydrates: 16g   Fats: 9g

30. Squash Black Bean Bowl

Preparation Time: 5 Minutes
Cooking Time: 30 Minutes
Servings: 4

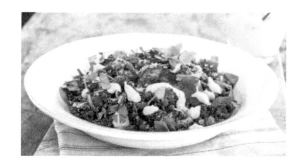

Ingredients:

- 1 large spaghetti squash, halved, seeded
- ⅓ Cup water (or 2 tbsp olive oil, rubbed on the inside of squash)
- Black bean filling
- One 15-oz can of black beans, emptied and rinsed 1 cup fire-roasted corn (or frozen sweet corn)
- 1 cup thinly sliced red cabbage
- 3 tbsp chopped green onion, green and white parts ¼ cup chopped fresh cilantro
- ½ lime, juiced or to taste
- Pepper and salt, to taste
- Avocado mash:
- 1 ripe avocado, mashed
- ½ lime, juiced or to taste
- ¼ tsp cumin
- Pepper and pinch of sea salt

Directions:

1. Preheat the oven to 400°F.
2. Chop the squash in part and scoop out the seeds with a spoon, like a pumpkin.
3. Fill the roasting pan with ⅓ cup of water. Lay the squash, cut side down, in the pan. Bake for 30 minutes until soft and tender.
4. While this is baking, mix all the ingredients for the black bean filling in a medium-sized bowl.
5. In a small dish, crush the avocado and blend in the ingredients for the avocado mash.
6. Eliminate the squash from the oven and let it cool for 5minutes. Scrape the squash with a fork so that it looks like spaghetti noodles. Then, fill it with black bean filling and top with avocado mash.
7. Serve and enjoy.

Nutrition:

Calories: 85   Fats: 0.5g   Carbohydrates: 6g   Protein: 4g

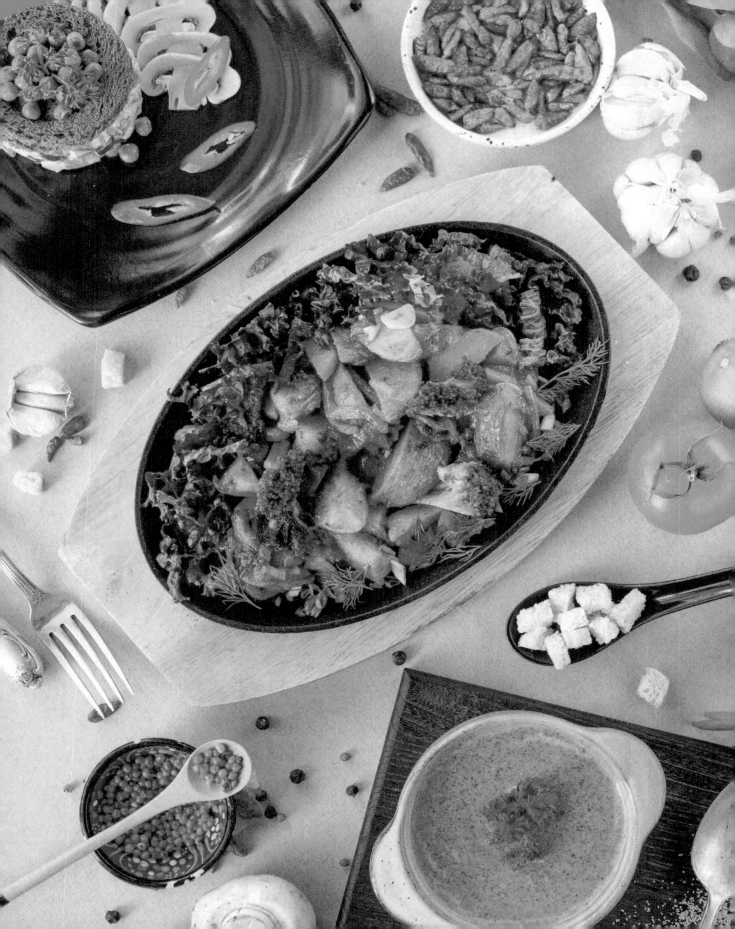

31.   Split Pea Pesto Stuffed Shells

Preparation time: 15 minutes

Cooking time: 60 minutes

Servings: 6

Nutrition

Calories: 82,   Protein 6g,

Fats 0 g,   Fiber 6g

Carbs 15 g,

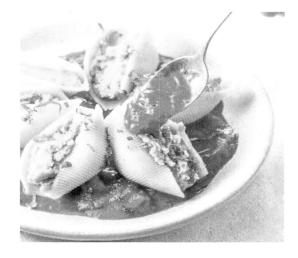

Ingredients

- 12 ounces jumbo pasta shells, whole grain, cooked
- Marinara sauce as needed for serving
- For the Split Pea Pesto:
- 1 cup green split peas
- ¼ cup basil leaves
- 1 teaspoon minced garlic
- 1 teaspoon of sea salt
- 2 tablespoons lemon juice
- 2 ¼ cups water, divided

Directions

1. Take a small saucepan, place it over high heat, add peas, pour in 2 cups water, and bring the beans to boil. Switch heat to a low level, simmer beans for 30 minutes, and when done, drain the beans then transfer them to a food processor.
2. Pour in remaining ingredients for the pesto and pulse until blended.
3. Take a baking dish, spread the marinara sauce in the bottom, then stuffed shell with prepared pesto, arrange them into the prepared baking dish, spread with some marinara sauce over the top and bake for 30 minutes until heated.
4. Garnish with basil and serve.

32. Coriander Okra and Kale

Preparation time: 10 minutes

Servings: 4

Cooking time: 20 minutes

Ingredients

- 2 tablespoons avocado oil
- 1 tablespoon mustard seeds
- 2 teaspoons ginger, grated
- 2 medium garlic cloves, chopped
- 1 pound okra, sliced
- ½ pound kale, torn
- 2 teaspoons coriander, ground
- 2 tablespoons sesame seeds, toasted
- Salt and black pepper to your taste

Directions

1. Heat up a pan with the oil over medium heat, add the ginger, garlic and
2. mustard seeds and sauté for 5 minutes.
3. Add the okra and the other ingredients, stir, cook over medium heat for 15
4. minutes, divide between plates and serve.

Nutrition:

Calories 120 g   Fat 6.4 g   Fiber 3 g   Carbs 10 g

Protein 4 g

33. Thai Peanut and Sweet Potato Buddha Bowl

Preparation time: 10 minutes

Cooking time: 20 minutes

Servings: 2

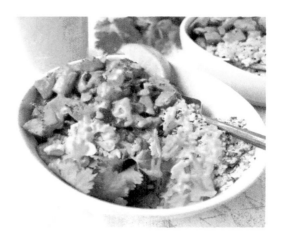

Ingredients

- 1 cup quinoa, cooked
- 4 cups sweet potato, peeled, small dice
- ½ cup carrots shredded
- ¼ cup cilantro
- 2 teaspoons minced garlic
- 2 teaspoons chopped rosemary
- 1 teaspoon salt
- 1 teaspoon ground cinnamon
- 1 teaspoon ground black pepper
- ¼ cup peanuts, chopped
- ¼ cup olive oil
- ½ cup Thai Peanut Sauce
- Ingredients For the Thai Peanut Sauce
- ¼ cup Thai red curry paste
- ¼ cup brown sugar
- 2 tablespoons soy sauce
- 1 tablespoon lime juice
- 1 ½ cups coconut milk
- 2 tablespoons apple cider vinegar
- cup peanut butter

Directions

- Place sweet potatoes in a baking dish, add garlic, drizzle with oil, sprinkle with salt, rosemary, black pepper, and cinnamon and bake for 20 minutes at 425°f until roasted.
- Meanwhile, prepare the peanut sauce, and for this, place all its ingredients in a food processor and pulse until smooth.
- When sweet potatoes have cooked, distribute them between 2 bowls along with peanuts, quinoa, cilantro, and carrots and then drizzle with sauce generously.
- Serve straight away.

Nutrition:

Calories: 202   Fats 1.3 g   Carbs 47 g   Protein 4 g

Fiber 7.4 g

34. Buffalo Cauliflower Tacos

Preparation time: 10 minutes

Servings: 4

Cooking time: 20 minutes

Ingredients For the Cauliflower:
- ½ head cauliflower, cut into florets
- 1 teaspoon garlic powder
- ¼ teaspoon ground black pepper
- 1 teaspoon red chili powder
- 4 teaspoons olive oil
- 3/4 cup buffalo sauce
- Ingredients For the Tacos:
- 1 medium head of romaine lettuce, chopped
- 8 flour tortillas
- 1 medium avocado, pitted, diced
- Vegan ranch as needed
- Chopped cilantro as needed

Directions
1. Place cauliflower florets in a bowl, add garlic powder, black pepper, red chili powder, olive oil, and ¼ cup buffalo sauce and toss until combined.
2. Spread cauliflower florets on a baking sheet in a single layer and cook for 20
3. minutes until roasted, flipping halfway.
4. When done, transfer cauliflower to a large bowl, then heat remaining buffalo sauce, add to cauliflower florets and toss until combined.
5. Assemble tacos and for this, top tortilla with cauliflower, lettuce, and avocado, drizzle with ranch dressing and then top with green onions.
6. Serve straight away.

Nutrition:

Calories: 250   Fats 9 g   Carbs 37 g   Protein 9 g

Fiber 5.4 g

35. Peanut vegetable noodle bowl

Preparation time: 10 minutes

Servings: 4

Cooking time: 10 minutes

Ingredients
- ½ cup thinly sliced bell pepper
- 8 oz. noodles
- 1 thin sliced carrot
- ½ thin sliced cucumber
- ½ cup chopped cilantro
- 1/3 cup chopped peanuts
- 1 chopped onion
- 2 tablespoons toasted sesame oil
- ¼ cup peanut butter
- 2 tablespoons pure maple syrup
- 1 tablespoon minced garlic and ginger
- 1 tablespoon apple cider vinegar

Directions
1. Cook the noodles by following the directions given on the package.
2. After cooking it, drain the water and rinse it with cold water and put it aside.
3. In a bowl, add peanut butter, sesame oil, vinegar, ginger, garlic, maples syrup, and soy sauce and combine it well.
4. In another bowl, add noodles and add all the remaining ingredients in it and serve.

Nutrition:

Calories 553   Carbs 74g   Protein 12g   Fats 24g

36. Meatball Sub

Preparation time: 10 minutes

Servings: 3

Cooking time: 22 minutes

Ingredients For the Meatballs:

- 1/3 cup sunflower seeds, ground
- 1 ½ cups cooked kidney beans
- ½ cup mushrooms, chopped
- ½ cup rolled oats
- ½ teaspoon minced garlic
- 1 small red onion, peeled, chopped
- 2/3 teaspoon salt
- 1 teaspoon dried oregano
- 1/3 teaspoon ground black pepper
- 1 teaspoon dried basil
- 1 teaspoon soy sauce
- 1 tablespoon olive oil
- 1 tablespoon tomato paste
- Ingredients For the Subs:
- 3 Italian sub rolls
- ¼ cup chopped parsley
- 2 cups marinara sauce
- 3 tablespoons grated vegan Parmesan

Directions

1. Place beans in a bowl, mash them with a fork and set aside until required.
2. Then place a medium pan over medium heat, add oil and when hot, add onions - cook for 3 minutes. Stir in garlic and mushrooms and cook for another 2 minutes.
3. Then stir in mashed beans, add oats, sunflower seeds, tomato paste, all the spices and soy sauce, stir until well combined, and shape the mixture into 14
4. meatballs.
5. Arrange meatballs onto a baking sheet lined with parchment paper and bake for 15 minutes at 350°f until cooked.
6. Sandwich the meatballs evenly between sub rolls, top with marinara, parmesan cheese, and parsley, and then serve.

Nutrition:

Calories: 404   Fats 14 g   Carbs 60 g   Protein 13 g

Fiber 10 g

37. Pumpkin buckwheat Penne

Preparation time: 10 minutes

Cooking time: 60 minutes

Servings: 4

Nutrition

Calories: 301   Protein 16.3 g

Fats 6.1 g   Fiber 6.3 g

Carbs 46.2 g

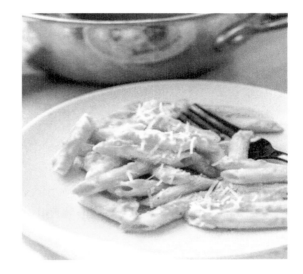

Ingredients

- ½ of medium white onion, sliced into wedges
- 2 cloves of garlic, unpeeled
- 1 cup cooked and mashed sugar pie pumpkin
- ½ cup unsalted cashews, soaked, drained
- ½ teaspoon of sea salt
- 1/3 teaspoon ground black pepper
- 5 fresh sage leaves
- 2 tablespoons olive oil and more as needed for drizzling 1 cup vegetable broth
- 16 ounces penne buckwheat pasta

Directions

1. Take a baking sheet, place onion, pumpkin and garlic on it, drizzle with oil, season with salt and black pepper, pierce pumpkin with a fork, cover the baking sheet and bake for 45 minutes until vegetables are very tender.
2. Then add sage in the last five minutes and after 45 minutes of baking, uncover the baking sheet and continue baking for 15 minutes.
3. When done, peel the pumpkin and add to the food processor along with remaining vegetables and ingredients (except for pasta) and puree until blended.
4. Place pasta in a pot, add half of the blended pumpkin mixture, stir until coated, and then stir in remaining pumpkin mixture and serve.

38.   White Bean and Mushroom Meatballs Subs

Preparation time: 15 minutes

Servings: 20

Cooking time: 30 minutes

Ingredients:

- 1 ¼ cups breadcrumbs
- 15 ounces cooked white beans
- 1 small white onion, peeled, diced
- 8 ounces button mushrooms, chopped
- 1 teaspoon minced garlic
- ½ teaspoon ground black pepper
- 1 teaspoon salt
- ½ teaspoon red chili flake
- 1 teaspoon oregano
- 1 lemon, juiced
- 1 tablespoon olive oil
- 2 tablespoons parsley, chopped
- Ingredients For the Subs:
- 15 ounces marinara sauce
- 20 sub rolls

Directions

1. Take a large skillet pan, place it over medium heat, add oil and when hot, add onion and cook for 5 minutes.
2. Then add garlic and mushrooms, cook for 2 minutes, add beans, season with salt, red chili flakes, oregano, and black pepper, stir in lemon juice and cook for 1 minute.
3. Transfer the mixture into the food processor, puree until smooth, add 1 cup crumbs and parsley and pulse until well combined.
4. Let the mixture stand for five minutes, shape the mixture into twenty meatballs, cover with remaining breadcrumbs until coated, and cook for 20
5. minutes until nicely browned on all sides.
6. Sandwich the meatballs in sub rolls, top with marinara sauce and serve.

Nutrition:

Calories			
	404Fats 14 g	Carbs 60 g	Protein 13 g
Fiber 10 g			

39. Sweet Potato Fries

Preparation time: 10 minutes

Servings: 4

Cooking time: 30 minutes

Ingredients

- 3 large, sweet potatoes
- ½ teaspoon sea salt
- ¼ teaspoon cayenne pepper
- 1 teaspoon cumin
- ¼ teaspoon paprika
- 1 tablespoon olive oil

Directions

1. Peel the potatoes, cut into wedges lengthwise, place them in a bowl, drizzle with oil and toss until combined.
2. Stir together remaining ingredients, sprinkle over sweet potatoes, spread the potatoes evenly on a baking sheet greased with oil and bake for 30 minutes at 400°f until done, tossing twice.
3. Serve straight away.

Nutrition:

Calories: 78   Fats 4 g   Carbs 11g   Protein 1 g,
Fiber 2g

40. Vegetarian Biryani

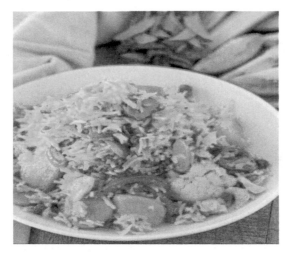

Preparation time: 10 minutes

Cooking time: 33 minutes

Servings: 6

Nutrition:

Calories: 385	Carbs 73.6 g,
Fats 6.8 g,	Protein 8.6 g
Fiber 5.5 g	

Ingredients

- 12 ounces chickpeas
- 2 cups rice, rinsed
- 1 large onion, peeled, sliced
- 2 cups sliced mixed veggies
- 1 ½ teaspoon minced garlic
- 1 tablespoon grated ginger
- 1 tablespoon cumin
- ½ teaspoon turmeric
- 1 tablespoon coriander
- 3/4 teaspoon salt
- 1 teaspoon cinnamon
- ½ teaspoon cardamom
- 1 bay leaf
- ½ cup raisins
- 2 tablespoons olive oil
- 1 teaspoon red chili powder
- 4 cups vegetable stock
- Ingredients For Garnishing:
- ¼ cup cashews
- ¼ cup chopped parsley

Directions

1. Take a large skillet pan, place it over medium-high heat, add oil and when hot, add onion and cook for 5 minutes.
2. Then add vegetables, ginger, and garlic, continue cooking for 5 minutes, reserve 1 cup of the mixture and set it aside.
3. Add bay leaf into the pan, stir in all the spices, cook for 1 minute, stir in rice and cook for a further 1 minute.
4. Season with salt, pour in the stock, then top with reserved vegetables, chickpeas and raisins, switch heat to a high level, and bring the mixture to simmer.
5. Then switch heat to a low level, cover the pan with a towel, place lid on top of it to seal the pan completely, and simmer for 20 minutes until all the liquid has soaked by the rice.
6. When done, fluff the rice with a fork, top with cilantro and cashews, and then serve.

41. Roasted Cauliflower

Preparation time: 10 minutes

Servings: 4

Cooking time: 1 hour and 20 minutes

Ingredients

- 1 medium head of cauliflower
- ½ teaspoon salt
- 1 teaspoon dried parsley
- 1 teaspoon dried dill
- 1 teaspoon dried mint
- 1 tablespoon zaatar spice
- 2 tablespoons olive oil, divided
- 1 cup of water

Directions

1. Trim the cauliflower, then slice from the bottom, drizzle it with 1 tablespoon oil, season with salt and zaatar spice, cover cauliflower with foil and bake for 55 minutes.
2. When done, uncover the cauliflower, drizzle with remaining oil and bake for 30 minutes until roasted, turning halfway.
3. Sprinkle with parsley, dill, and milk and serve cauliflower with lemon wedges and tahini sauce.

Nutrition:

Calories: 127   Fats 8 g   Protein 5 g   Fiber 5.1 g

Carbs 13 g

42.   Chinese Eggplant with Szechuan Sauce

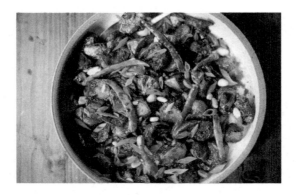

Preparation time: 10 minutes

Cooking time: 25 minutes

Servings: 4

Ingredients

- 1 ½ pounds eggplant
- 2 teaspoons minced garlic
- 2 teaspoons grated ginger
- 2 tablespoons cornstarch
- 2 teaspoons salt
- 4 tablespoons peanut oil
- 10 dried red chilies
- Ingredients For the Szechuan Sauce:
- 1 teaspoon Szechuan peppercorns, toasted, crushed
- ½ teaspoon five-spice
- 1 tablespoon mirin
- 3 tablespoons brown sugar
- 1 teaspoon red chili flakes
- ¼ cup soy sauce

- 1 tablespoon rice vinegar
- 1 tablespoon sesame oil

Directions

1. Cut eggplant into bite-size pieces, place them in a large bowl, cover them with water, stir in salt and let them stand for 15 minutes.
2. Prepare the Szechuan sauce and for this, place all its ingredients in a small bowl except for Szechuan peppercorns and whisk until combined and set aside until required.
3. Pat dry eggplant with paper towels, sprinkle with corn starch and then fry them in a single layer over medium heat for 10 minutes until golden brown.
4. When eggplants are done, transfer them to a plate, add some more oil into the pan, add garlic and ginger and cook for 2 minutes.
5. Add Szechuan peppercorns and prepared sauce, stir until combined and simmer for 20 seconds.
6. Return eggplant pieces into the pan, toss until mixed, cook for 1 minute and then garnish with green onions.
7. Serve straight away.

Nutrition

Calories: 323   Fats 22 g   Carbs 30 g   Protein 6 g   Fiber 7.4 g

43. Ramen with Miso Shiitake

Preparation time: 10 minutes

Cooking time: 35 minutes

Servings: 4

Ingredients For Ramen Broth:
- 1 large white onion, peeled, diced
- 1/3 teaspoon ground black pepper
- ½ cup dried Shiitake Mushrooms, chopped
- 2 tablespoons white miso paste
- 1 teaspoon minced garlic
- 2 tablespoons olive oil
- 1/8 cup mirin
- 4 cups vegetable stock
- 4 cups of water

Ingredients For the Ramen:
- 8 ounces cubed tofu, crispy as needed
- 8 ounces cooked ramen noodles as needed
- Sautéed Bok choy as needed
- Fresh spinach as needed
- Shredded carrots as needed
- Roasted winter squash as needed
- Roasted cauliflower as needed
- Roasted carrots as needed
- Roasted sweet potato as needed
- Sautéed mushrooms as needed
- Smoked mushrooms as needed
- Pickled radish as needed
- Mix herbs as needed

Ingredients For Garnish:
- Scallions as needed
- Sesame seeds as needed
- Sriracha as needed
- Sesame oil as needed

Directions
1. Prepare the broth and for this, place a pot over medium-high heat, add 1tablespoon oil and when hot, add onion and cook for 3 minutes. Switch heat to medium level, stir in garlic, cook for 1 minute, then add remaining ingredients for the broth and simmer for 30 minutes until done. Distribute all the ingredients for ramen evenly between 4 bowls, then pour in broth and top with garnishing ingredients. Serve straight away.

Nutrition:

Calories: 408	Fats 14 g	Carbs 60 g	Protein 14 g	Fiber 4.3 g

44. Butternut Squash Linguine

Preparation time: 10 minutes

Cooking time: 35 minutes

Servings: 4

Ingredients

- 1 medium white onion, peeled, chopped
- 3 cups diced butternut squash, peeled, deseeded
- 1 teaspoon minced garlic
- ½ teaspoon salt
- ⅛ teaspoon red pepper flakes
- ¼ teaspoon ground black pepper
- 1 tablespoon chopped sage
- 2 tablespoons olive oil
- 2 cups vegetable broth
- 12 ounces linguine, whole grain, cooked

Directions

1. Take a large skillet pan, place it over medium heat, add oil and when hot, add sage and cook for 3 minutes until crispy.
2. Transfer sage to a bowl, sprinkle with some salt and set aside until required.
3. Add onion, squash pieces, and garlic into the pan, season with salt, red pepper and black pepper, stir until mixed and cook for 10 minutes.
4. Pour in broth, stir, and bring the mixture to boil, then switch heat to medium-low level and simmer for 20 minutes.
5. When done, remove the pan from heat, puree by using an immersion blender until smooth, taste to adjust seasoning and return it into the pan.
6. Heat the pan over medium heat, add cooked pasta, toss until well coated and cook for 2 minutes until hot.
7. Serve straight away.

Nutrition:

Calories: 380   Fats 9 g   Carbs 68.4 g   Protein 10.7 g   Fiber 10.8 g

45. Sweet Potato and Bean Burgers

Preparation time: 10 minutes

Cooking time: 50 minutes

Servings: 8

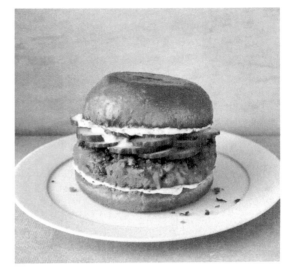

Ingredients

- 1 cup oats, old-fashioned, ground
- 1 ½ pounds sweet potatoes
- 1 cup cooked millet
- 15 ounces cooked black beans
- ½ cup cilantro, chopped
- ½ small red onion, peeled, diced
- ½ teaspoon salt
- 1 teaspoon chipotle powder
- 2 teaspoons cumin powder
- ½ teaspoon cayenne powder
- 1 teaspoon red chili powder
- 2 tablespoons olive oil
- 8 hamburger buns, whole-wheat, toasted

Directions

1. Prepare sweet potatoes, and for this, slice them lengthwise and roast for 40
2. minutes at 400°f, cut side up.
3. Prepare the burgers and for this, place all the ingredients in the bowl, except for oil and buns, stir until combined, and then shape the mixture into eight patties.
4. Take a skillet pan, place it over medium heat, add oil and when hot, add patties and cook for 4 minutes per side until browned.
5. Sandwich patties between buns, and serve

Nutrition:

Calories: 255 g   Fats 12.7   Carbs 29 g   Protein 10 g   Fiber 7.3 g

46.   Butternut Squash Chipotle Chili

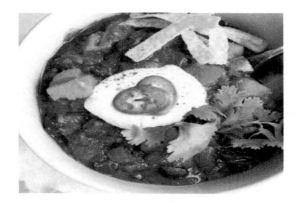

Preparation time: 10 minutes

Cooking time: 60 minutes

Servings: 4

Ingredients

- 3 cups cooked black beans
- 2 avocados, pitted, peeled, diced
- 1 small butternut squash, peeled, ½-inch cubed
- 1 medium red onion, peeled, chopped
- 2 teaspoons minced garlic
- 1 tablespoon chopped chipotle pepper in adobo
- 14 ounces diced tomatoes with the juices
- 2 medium red bell peppers, chopped
- ¼ teaspoon ground cinnamon
- 1 tablespoon red chili powder
- 1 ½ teaspoon salt
- 1 teaspoon ground cumin
- 1 bay leaf
- 2 tablespoons olive oil
- 2 cups vegetable broth
- 3 corn tortillas

Directions

1. Cook onion, squash, and bell pepper in oil in a large stockpot placed over medium heat for 5 minutes.
2. Switch heat to medium-low level, add peppers, garlic, cumin, cinnamon, and chili powder, stir until mixed and cook for 30 seconds.
3. Then add remaining ingredients, except for tortilla, stir until combined and cook for 1 hour until done, adjusting the taste halfway.
4. Meanwhile, prepare the tortilla chips and for this, cut tortillas into 2 inches by ¼ inch strips, place a skillet pan over medium heat, add oil and when hot, toss in tortilla strips, sprinkle with some salt and cook for 7 minutes until golden.
5. When done, transfer tortilla chips to a plate lined with paper towels and serve with cooked chili.

Nutrition:

Calories: 202   Fats 1.4 g   Carbs 41 g   Protein 10.2 g   Fiber 13.5 g

47. Romaine Lettuce and Radicchios Mix

Preparation time: 6 minutes

Servings: 4

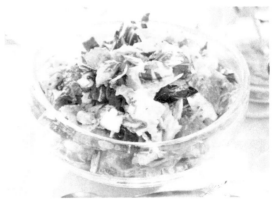

Ingredients

- 2 tablespoons olive oil
- A pinch of salt and black pepper
- 2 spring onions, chopped
- 3 tablespoons Dijon mustard
- Juice of 1 lime
- ½ cup basil, chopped
- 4 cups romaine lettuce heads, chopped
- 3 radicchios, sliced

Directions

1. In a salad bowl, mix the lettuce with the spring onions and the other ingredients, toss and serve.

Nutrition:

Calories 87   Carbs 1 g   Fiber 1 g   Protein 2 g

Fats 2 g

48. Greek Salad

Preparation Time: 15 Minutes

Cooking Time: 15 Minutes

Servings: 5

Ingredients For Dressing

- ½ teaspoon black pepper
- ¼ teaspoon salt
- ½ teaspoon oregano
- 1 tablespoon garlic powder
- 2 tablespoons Balsamic
- 1/3 cup olive oil
- Ingredients For Salad
- ½ cup sliced black olives
- ½ cup chopped parsley, fresh
- 1 small red onion, thin sliced
- 1 cup cherry tomatoes, sliced
- 1 bell pepper, yellow, chunked
- 1 cucumber, peeled, quarter and slice
- 4 cups chopped romaine lettuce
- ½ teaspoon salt
- 2 tablespoons olive oil

Directions

1. In a small bowl, blend all the ingredients for the dressing and let this set in the refrigerator while you make the salad.
2. To assemble the salad, mix together all the ingredients in a large-sized bowl and toss the veggies gently but thoroughly to mix.
3. Serve the salad with the dressing in amounts as desired

Nutrition:

| Calories 234 | Fat 16.1 g | Protein 5 g | Carbs 48 g |

49. Roasted Pepper Pasta Salad

Preparation time: 30 minutes

Cooking Time: 8/10 minutes

Servings: 4

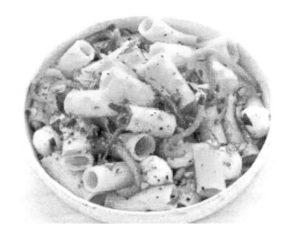

Ingredients
- 6 ounces whole-wheat penne
- ½ teaspoon black pepper
- ½ teaspoon salt
- Garlic, 1 clove peeled and minced
- 1 ½ teaspoons lemon juice
- 1 tablespoon olive oil
- 2 tablespoons basil, fresh
- 2 tablespoons capers, chopped
- ½ cup scallions, chop finely
- 17 ounces roasted red peppers, rinsed and sliced

Directions
1. Use the directions on the package to cook the pasta.
2. When it is done, drain it well and refrigerate the pasta until it is cool to cold as preferred.
3. When the pasta has cooled to your liking, then mix the scallions, capers, and red peppers in a medium-sized bowl with the lemon juice, garlic, salt, black pepper, oil, and basil.
4. Toss the ingredients well so that all are well coated, and the flavors are mixed well. Add in the cooked noodles and toss well.

Nutrition:

Calories 198   Carbs 39g   Fiber 6g   Protein 8g

Fat 5g

50. Salad Niçoise

Preparation time: 45 minutes

Servings: 4

Ingredients For Dressing:
- 2 tablespoons lemon juice
- 1 tablespoon water
- Salt, 1 quarter teaspoon
- ¼ teaspoon black pepper
- 1 tablespoons olive oil
- 1 clove garlic, minced
- Ingredients For Salad:
- ½ cup French-style green beans
- 1 tablespoon olive oil
- ½ teaspoon salt
- ½ teaspoon black pepper
- 1 large head bibb lettuce
- 2 tablespoons basil, dried
- ¼ cup black olives, pitted
- Red potato wedges, 2 cups
- ½ cup red onion, thin sliced
- 1 cup grape tomatoes

Directions
1. Use a medium-sized bowl to mix all the dressing ingredients together, and then refrigerate.
2. Cook the green beans for 2 minutes in water and then drain them well.
3. Set a large skillet over medium-high heat to warm 1 tablespoon of the olive oil and cook the potatoes for five minutes on each side, stirring them well and often.
4. Arrange the torn leaves of the Bibb lettuce evenly on 4 plates and sprinkle them with the basil.
5. Divide the onions, green beans, potatoes, olives, and tomatoes evenly over the 4 plates on top of the lettuce.
6. Serve the salads with the chilled dressing.

Nutrition

Calories 213	Fiber 4.8g	Carbs 20.8g	Protein 4.5 g
Fat 5.4g			

51. Tomato Salad

Preparation time: 15 minutes

Servings: 6

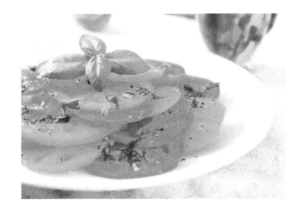

Ingredients

- ¼ cup basil leaves, chopped fresh
- 1 cup yellow tomatoes, sliced thinly
- 1 cup red tomatoes, sliced thinly
- 2 tablespoons chives, chop finely
- 1-pint grape tomatoes, halved
- 1 teaspoon black pepper
- ½ teaspoon salt
- 2 tablespoons balsamic vinegar
- ¼ cup olive oil

Directions

1. Mix in a medium-sized bowl the salt, pepper, balsamic vinegar, and the olive oil until well blended.
2. Put the tomatoes in this mix and toss them gently to coat them well.
3. Sprinkle the top of the mix with the chives and the fresh basil.

Nutrition:

Calories 105   Fat 9.5g   Carbs 6g   Protein 1g

52. Cauliflower Sweet Potato Salad

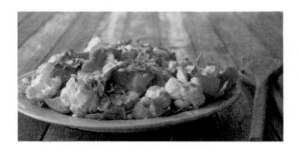

Preparation time: 20 minutes

Cooking time: 30 minutes

Servings: 8

Ingredients

- ½ cup cranberries, dried
- 8 cups lettuce, any variety, torn
- 1 tablespoon balsamic vinegar
- 1 teaspoon black pepper
- 1 teaspoon salt
- 7 tablespoons olive oil, divided
- 1 small head cauliflower, broken into florets
- 1 ½ pound sweet potatoes, cut into ½ inch wide wedges

Directions

1. Heat the oven to 425°f. Mix together in a medium-sized bowl the cauliflower florets and the sweet potato wedges with the pepper, salt, and tablespoons of the olive oil. Spread these out on a cookie sheet and bake them for thirty minutes and then let them cool slightly.
2. During the time that the veggies are roasting, mix the balsamic vinegar and the remainder of the olive oil in a large bowl.
3. Then add in the dried cranberries, lettuce, and the cooled roasted veggies.
4. Toss this mixture well to coat all pieces and serve immediately.

Nutrition:

Calories 150   Fiber 3 g   Carbs 11 g   Protein 5 g

Fat 12 g

53. Tropical Style Radicchio Salad

Preparation time: 15 minutes

Servings: 6

Ingredients

- ½ teaspoon black pepper
- ½ teaspoon salt
- 2 tablespoons orange juice
- ¼ cup basil leaves, chopped, firmly packed
- 2 cups pineapple, fresh, finely chop
- 2 tablespoons coconut oil
- 2 medium heads radicchio, cut into quarters from top to the bottom

Directions

1. Heat the oven to 450°f.
2. Use the coconut oil to brush both sides of the pieces of radicchio.
3. Bake the radicchio for ten minutes, turning over after five minutes. Allow the radicchio to cool. When it has cooled to room temperature, slice it very thinly, to look like chopped cabbage, and then place it in a large-sized bowl.
4. Add in the pepper, salt, orange juice, basil, and pineapple and toss the ingredients gently but well to mix them together and coat all pieces well.
5. You can serve it right away or keep it in the refrigerator for no more than 1 day.

Nutrition:

Calories 40   Carbs 25 g   Fat 2 g   Fiber 20 g

54. Winter Vegetable Salad

Preparation time: 10 minutes

Cooking time: 40 minutes

Servings: 3

Ingredients For Salad:

- 4 cups salad mixed greens, packed
- 2 tablespoons balsamic vinegar
- 1 tablespoon olive oil
- 2 tablespoons basil, dried
- 1 tablespoon coriander, dried
- 1 teaspoon rosemary
- 1 teaspoon marjoram
- 2 tablespoons parsley, fresh, chop finely
- 1 teaspoon black pepper
- ½ teaspoon salt

Ingredients For Roasted Vegetables:

- 1 tablespoon olive oil
- ½ teaspoon salt
- 1 teaspoon black pepper
- 2 parsnips
- 2 carrots
- 10 baby red potatoes
- 1 small butternut squash
- 1 red onion

Directions

1. Heat the oven to 400°f.
2. Wash the potatoes, carrots, and parsnips and dry them with a paper towel.
3. Wipe off the squash and the onion and peel them.
4. Chop all the vegetables into bite-sized chunks. Place all the chunks into a large-sized bowl with the pepper, salt, and olive oil.
5. Toss all the vegetables in the bowl with the olive oil until they are well coated. Spread out the oiled veggies on a cookie sheet and bake them in the oven for forty minutes.
6. While the veggies are roasting, you can mix up the dressing for the salad.
7. Mix the balsamic vinegar with the olive oil and all the pepper, salt, and herbs.
8. When you take the vegetables from the oven, divide them into servings and pour the dressing over the top of the veggie servings as personally desired.

Nutrition:

Calories 483   Fat 12 g   Carbs 85 g   Fiber 17 g
Protein 11 g

55. Vegan Cobb Salad

Preparation time: 20 Minutes

Servings: 4

Ingredients For Vinaigrette:
- ½ cup olive oil
- ½ teaspoon black pepper
- ½ teaspoon salt
- 1 teaspoon garlic, minced,
- 1 tablespoon Dijon mustard
- 1/3 cup balsamic vinegar
- Ingredients For Salad:
- 2 avocados, sliced
- Tempeh (soybean) bacon
- ½ cup red onion, chopped
- ½ cup corn, thawed frozen or fresh
- 1 cup carrots, grated
- 1 large cucumber, peeled and chopped
- 1 cup grape tomatoes, cut in half
- 2 fifteen-ounce cans chickpeas, drained and rinsed 12 cups greens – chopped romaine, spring mix, or baby spinach or a mix of these

Directions
1. In a glass jar or a small bowl, mix well all the ingredients for the vinaigrette dressing and put it in the refrigerator until you are ready to serve the salad.
2. Use the directions on the package to cook the tempeh bacon.
3. Divide the greens between 4 salad plates or bowls.
4. Arrange on top of the greens equal amounts of the tempeh bacon, red onion, corn, carrots, cucumber, tomatoes, and chickpeas.
5. Lay the slices of avocado over the ingredients on top of the lettuce and drizzle on the amount of the salad dressing you prefer.

Nutrition:

Calories 385   Fat 11 g   Fiber 20 g   Carbs 54 g   Protein 19 g

56. Greek Style Spring Soup

Preparation time: 10 minutes

Cooking time: 25 minutes

Servings: 5

Ingredients

- Chives, fresh minced for garnish
- 2 tablespoons olive oil
- 6 cups vegetable broth
- ½ teaspoon salt
- 1 teaspoon black pepper
- 1 teaspoon turmeric
- 1 teaspoon rosemary
- 1 bay leaf
- 1 small onion, diced
- ½ cup dill, fresh, chopped
- 1 cup carrots, diced
- 1 cup asparagus, chopped
- 2 tablespoons lemon juice
- ½ cup brown rice

Directions

1. Use a large pot for cooking the onions for five minutes.
2. Pour in ½ cup of the dill with the bay leaf and vegetable broth and boil.
3. Mix in the rice and lower the heat and simmer for fifteen more minutes. Put in the carrots and asparagus and simmer ten more minutes.
4. Remove the bay leaf and add the lemon juice and the rest of the seasonings.
5. Stir well and serve, garnishing each serving with the remaining fresh dill.

Nutrition:

Calories 341   Fat 9.7 g   Carbs 30 g   Fiber 4 g

Protein 12 g

57. Roasted Red Pepper and Tomato Soup

Preparation time: 10 minutes

Cooking time: 45 minutes

Servings: 4

Ingredients

- 2 red bell peppers, seeded and cut in half
- 1 tomato, cored and halved
- ¼ teaspoon cayenne pepper
- 2 tablespoons olive oil
- 2 tablespoons garlic, minced
- ¼ teaspoon paprika, ground
- ½ teaspoon Italian seasoning
- ¼ cup parsley, fresh, chopped
- 2 tablespoons tomato paste
- 2 cups vegetable broth
- 1 teaspoon black pepper
- ½ teaspoon salt
- 1 medium onion, cut in quarters

Directions

1. Heat oven to 400°f. In a bowl, toss the onion, tomatoes, garlic, and red pepper with the salt, pepper, and olive oil.
2. Lay the veggies on a baking pan and bake for forty-five minutes.
3. Heat the vegetable broth and add in the roasted vegetables to the broth, then puree the soup using a blender and then put it back in the pot just until it is warm, stirring well.

Nutrition:

Calories 150   Fat 3.2 g   Carbs 14.4 g   Fiber 3.3 g
Protein 3.3 g

58. Zucchini Soup

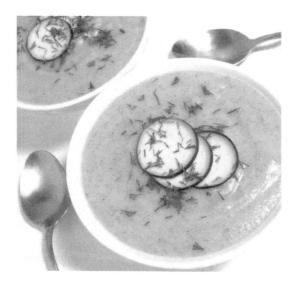

Preparation time: 15 minutes

Cooking time: 30 minutes

Servings: 8

Ingredients

- 2 pounds Zucchini, sliced thinly
- 1/3 cup basil, fresh
- ½ teaspoon salt
- 1 teaspoon turmeric
- ½ teaspoon thyme
- 1 teaspoon rosemary
- 1 teaspoon black pepper
- 4 cups vegetable broth
- 2 tablespoons garlic, minced
- 2 tablespoons olive oil
- 1 medium onion, diced

Directions

1. Cook the garlic, zucchini, and onion for five minutes in hot oil stirring often.
2. Stir in the vegetable broth and let this simmer for 15 minutes. Mix in salt and
3. pepper and all the spices and then blend the soup in a blender until creamy.
4. Return to stove just until warm.

Nutrition:

Calories 79   Fat 4.9 g   Carbs 28.8 g   Fiber 2.4 g
Protein 1.6 g

Preparation time: 20 minutes

Cooking time: 1 hour 10 minutes

Servings: 8

Ingredients

- 1 head cabbage, remove core and chop
- ½ teaspoon thyme, crushed
- 2 stalks celery, sliced thinly
- 2 carrots, sliced thinly
- 1 bay leaf
- ½ teaspoon salt
- 28ounce can crushed tomatoes
- 8ounce can tomato sauce
- 15ounce can with liquid red beans
- 6 cups water
- 1 onion, chopped
- ½ cup wild rice, uncooked
- 1 tablespoon olive oil

Directions

1. Cook the onion in hot olive oil in a large skillet for five minutes. Stir in the water.
2. Add in the beans, rice, crushed tomatoes, celery, tomato sauce, carrots, and cabbage and mix this together well. Mix in bay leaf, salt, and thyme.
3. Boil soup for 1 minute, and then lower the heat, simmering for 1 hour.
4. Remove the bay leaf and serve.

Nutrition:

Calories 404   Fat 10.6 g   Carbs 37.4 g   Fiber 9.8 g
Protein 20.3 g

CHAPTER 8

60. Tuscany Vegetable Soup

Preparation time: 15 minutes

Cooking time: 30 minutes

Servings: 8

Ingredients

- Parsley, fresh chopped for garnish
- 1 medium yellow onion, diced
- 2 tablespoons garlic, minced
- ½ teaspoon salt
- 1 teaspoon marjoram
- ½ teaspoon thyme
- 1 teaspoon black pepper
- 1 tablespoon basil, ground
- 2 cups kale, chopped
- 2 tablespoons tomato paste
- ½ cup celery, chopped
- ½ cup carrot, chopped
- 6 cups vegetable broth
- 2 large tomatoes, diced small
- 1 medium zucchini, peeled and chopped
- 1 tablespoon olive oil

Directions

1. Fry the garlic and the onion in the heated olive oil in a soup pot for two minutes. Then add in the carrots, celery, and the zucchini and cook for ten more minutes while stirring frequently.
2. Mix in well the tomatoes, marjoram, thyme, pepper, and salt and cook for 2
3. more minutes.
4. Pour in the vegetable broth and the tomato paste, mix well, and bring the
5. whole mix to a boil.
6. Turn the heat lower and let the mix simmer for 15 minutes.
7. Stir in the basil and the parsley, then remove the pot from the heat and let the soup sit for ten minutes.
8. Garnish with fresh parsley and serve.

Nutrition:

Calories 225   Carbs 12 g   Protein 17 g   Fat 6 g

61. Creamy Mushroom Soup

Preparation time: 1 hour

Cooking time: 30 minutes

Servings: 2

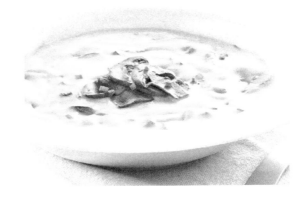

Ingredients

- 1 cup cashews, raw
- ½ teaspoon thyme
- ½ teaspoon white pepper
- 1 teaspoon salt
- 2 cups vegetable broth
- 1 tablespoon garlic, minced
- 1 shallot, chopped
- ½ pound cremini mushrooms, chopped
- 2 tablespoons olive oil

Directions

1. Let the raw cashews soak for thirty minutes in 6 cups of water that has been boiled.
2. Scoop out the cashews and save the water. Put ¼ cup of the water in a blender with the cashews and blend until creamy.
3. Drop-in a few more drops of water at a time if needed for a smooth consistency. Fry the garlic, shallot, and mushrooms in hot olive oil for ten minutes, stirring often.
4. Stir in the thyme, pepper, salt, and vegetable broth and mix all this well.
5. Let it simmer for five minutes and then add in the cashew cream (from the blender). Stir the soup until well mixed and serve. Garnish with some fresh parsley if you like.

Nutrition:

Calories 171   Fat 12.7 g   Carbs 8.8 g   Fiber 1 g
Protein 5.4 g

62. Coconut Lemon Lentil Soup

Preparation time: 10 minutes

Cooking time: 45 minutes

Servings: 6

Ingredients

- Cilantro or parsley, fresh, for garnish
- ¼ teaspoon red pepper flakes, crushed
- ½ teaspoon salt
- 1 teaspoon black pepper
- 1/3 cup coconut milk, full fat
- 2 tablespoons lemon juice
- ¼ cup tomato paste
- 2 cups red lentils
- 4 cups water
- 4 cups vegetable broth
- ½ teaspoon coriander
- 1 ½ teaspoons cumin
- 1 ½ teaspoons paprika
- 2 carrots, chopped
- 2 celery stalks, chopped
- 1 tablespoon garlic, minced
- 2 tablespoons coconut oil

Directions

1. Fry the onion in the hot oil in a large pot for two minutes.
2. Add in the garlic and cook for another minute.
3. Mix in the coriander, cumin, paprika, carrots, and celery and fry this for five minutes, stirring often.
4. Then add in the tomato paste, lentils, water, and broth and mix well.
5. Let this mixture come to a boil and then reduce the heat and let it simmer for forty to forty-five minutes or until the lentils are tender.
6. Then mix in the salt, pepper, coconut milk, and lemon juice and stir.
7. Top each serving with fresh parsley or cilantro as desired.

Nutrition:

Calories 161   Fat 7 g   Carbs 19 g   Fiber 15.8 g
Protein 13.2 g

63. Apple and Butternut Squash Soup

Preparation time: 10 minutes

Cooking time: 1 hour 20 minutes

Servings: 4

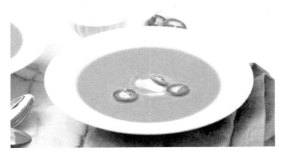

Ingredients

- 5 pounds (2 medium sized) butternut squash with seeds removed 1 large apple, any crisp variety like granny smith, cored, peeled, chopped 1 teaspoon salt
- 1 cup coconut milk
- 4 cups vegetable broth
- 1 tablespoon cinnamon, ground
- 1 cup carrot, chopped
- 1 large yellow onion, chopped
- 2 teaspoons olive oil

Directions

1. Heat oven to 425°f. Brush olive oil on each squash half and place inside down on a cookie sheet. Bake the squash for 1 hour. Let them cool for ten minutes.
2. While they are cooling warm the other teaspoon of olive oil and fry the onions, carrots, and apples for ten minutes, then add in the cinnamon, stir
3. well and remove from the heat.
4. Take the flesh of the squash out and put it in the pot. Mix in the vegetable broth and bring this mixture to a boil over medium-high heat, then simmer over a lower heat for twenty minutes. Stir in the salt and cinnamon. Then blend the soup ingredients in small batches until all of it is smooth and creamy.

Nutrition:

Calories 116   Fat 15 g   Carbs 28.7 g   Fiber 4.7 g

Protein 2.8 g

64. Quinoa Vegetables Soup

Preparation time: 15 minutes

Cooking time: 20 minutes

Servings: 8

Ingredients

- 2 tablespoons parsley
- 1 cup quinoa, uncooked, rinsed
- 1 teaspoon black pepper
- 2 tablespoons lemon juice
- 1 teaspoon salt
- 2 cups red cabbage, shredded
- 1 cup broccoli florets
- 1 bunch kale, chopped and stems removed
- 2 bay leaves
- 4 cups vegetable broth
- 1 teaspoon oregano, dried
- ½ teaspoon thyme, dried
- 2 stalks celery, diced
- 2 carrots, peeled and diced
- 1 red onion, diced
- 2 tablespoons garlic, minced
- 1 tablespoon olive oil

Directions

1. Use a Dutch oven or another large soup pot to warm the olive oil.
2. Stir in the celery, onion, and carrots and fry for 4 minutes.
3. Add in the oregano and thyme and mix well. Add in the water, bay leaves, and vegetable broth and bring the mix to a boil.
4. Stir in the quinoa and let the soup simmer for 15 minutes.
5. Add in the cabbage, broccoli, and kale and cook for five more minutes, stirring occasionally.
6. Blend in the pepper, salt, and lemon juice and serve.

Nutrition:

Calories 161   Fat 3.7 g   Carbs 27.1 g   Fiber 4.7 g
Protein 5.6 g

65. Mexican Style Vegetable Soup

Preparation time: 15 minutes

Cooking time: 35 minutes

Servings: 6

Ingredients

- ½ cup cilantro, chopped
- 2 tablespoons lime juice
- 2 cups corn, frozen or canned
- 1 teaspoon salt
- 1 teaspoon black pepper
- 1 teaspoon cumin, ground
- 1 teaspoon oregano, dried
- 1 red bell pepper, diced
- 1 cup green beans, frozen or canned
- 1 medium zucchini, chopped into bite-sized chunks
- 15ounce can diced tomatoes with green chilies, canned 5 cups vegetable broth
- 2 tablespoons garlic, minced
- 2 tablespoons olive oil
- 2 carrots, peeled and diced
- 1 yellow onion, peeled and diced

Directions

1. Over medium-high heat warm the olive oil in a large pot.
2. Fry the carrots and onions for two minutes.
3. Stir in the garlic and cook for 2 more minutes.
4. Mix in the zucchini, bell pepper, green beans, tomatoes, vegetables broth, pepper, salt, cumin, and oregano.
5. Mix all these together well and bring the mix to a full boil.
6. Simmer the soup over a lower heat for twenty to 25 minutes until all the vegetables are soft.
7. Mix in the cilantro, lime juice, and corn and cook for five more minutes and serve.

Nutrition:

Calories 103   Carbs 17.6 g   Fiber 3.9 g   Protein 2.8 g
Fat 3.1 g

66. Cream of Mushroom Soup

Preparation time: 5 minutes

Cooking time: 12 minutes

Servings: 6

Ingredients

- 1 medium white onion, peeled, chopped
- 16 ounces button mush rooms, sliced
- 1 ½ teaspoon minced garlic
- ¼ cup all-purpose flour
- ½ teaspoon ground black pepper
- 1 teaspoon dried thyme
- ¼ teaspoon nutmeg
- ½ teaspoon salt
- 2 tablespoons vegan butter
- 4 cups vegetable broth
- 1 ½cups coconut milk, unsweetened

Directions

1. Take a large pot, place it over medium-high heat, add butter and when it melts, add onions and garlic, stir in garlic and cook for 5 minutes until softened and nicely brown.
2. Then sprinkle flour over vegetables, continue cooking for 1 minute, then add remaining ingredients, stir until mixed and simmer for 5 minutes until thickened. Serve straight away

Nutrition:

Calories: 120   Carbs 12 g   Protein 6 g   Fiber 6 g
Fats 7 g

67. Cauliflower and Horseradish Soup

Preparation time: 5 minutes
Cooking time: 20 minutes
Servings: 4

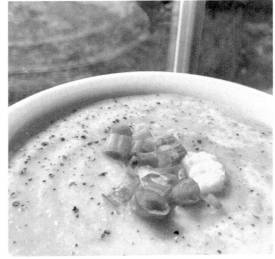

Ingredients
- 2 medium potatoes, peeled, chopped
- 1 medium cauliflower, florets and stalk chopped
- 1 medium white onion, peeled, chopped
- 1 teaspoon minced garlic
- 2/3 teaspoon salt
- 1/3 teaspoon ground black pepper
- 4 teaspoons horseradish sauce
- 1 teaspoon dried thyme
- 3 cups vegetable broth
- 1 cup coconut milk, unsweetened

Directions
1. Place all the vegetables in a large pan, place it over medium-high heat, add thyme, pour in broth and milk and bring the mixture to boil. Then switch heat
2. to medium level, simmer the soup for 15 minutes and remove the pan from heat.
3. Puree the soup by using an immersion blender until smooth, season with salt and black pepper, and serve straight away.

Nutrition:

Calories: 160   Carbs 31 g   Protein 6 g   Fiber 6 g
Fats 2.6 g

68. Curry Lentil Soup

Preparation time: 5 minutes

Cooking time: 40 minutes

Servings: 6

Ingredients

- 1 cup brown lentils
- 1 medium white onion, peeled, chopped
- 28 ounces diced tomatoes
- 1 ½ teaspoon minced garlic
- 1 inch of ginger, grated
- 3 cups vegetable broth
- ½ teaspoon salt
- 2 tablespoons curry powder
- 1 teaspoon cumin
- ½ teaspoon cayenne
- 1 tablespoon olive oil
- 1 ½ cups coconut milk, unsweetened
- ¼ cup chopped cilantro

Directions

1. Take a soup pot, place it over medium-high heat, add oil and when hot, add onion, stir in garlic and ginger and cook for 5 minutes until golden brown.
2. Then add all the ingredients except for milk and cilantro, stir until mixed and simmer for 25 minutes until lentils have cooked. When done, stir in milk, cook for 5 minutes until thoroughly heated and then garnish the soup with cilantro. Serve straight away

Nutrition:

Calories: 269   Carbs 26 g   Protein 10 g   Fiber 10 g
Fats 15 g

69. Chickpea Noodle Soup

Preparation time: 5 minutes
Cooking time: 18 minutes
Servings: 6

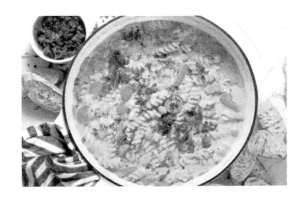

Ingredients

- 1 cup cooked chickpeas
- 8 ounces rotini noodles, whole-wheat
- 4 celery stalks, sliced
- 2 medium white onions, peeled, chopped
- 4 medium carrots, peeled, sliced
- 2 teaspoons minced garlic
- 8 sprigs of thyme
- 1 teaspoon salt
- 1/3 teaspoon ground black pepper
- 1 bay leaf
- 2 tablespoons olive oil
- 2 quarts of vegetable broth
- ¼ cup chopped fresh parsley

Directions

1. Take a large pot, place it over medium heat, add oil and when hot, add all the vegetables, stir in garlic, thyme and bay leaf and cook for 5 minutes until vegetables are golden and sauté.
2. Then pour in broth stir and bring the mixture to boil.
3. Add chickpeas and noodles into boiling soup, continue cooking for 8 minutes until noodles are tender, and then season soup with salt and black pepper.
4. Garnish with parsley and serve straight away

Nutrition:

Calories: 260   Carbs 44 g   Protein 7 g   Fiber 4 g
Fats 5 g

CHAPTER 8

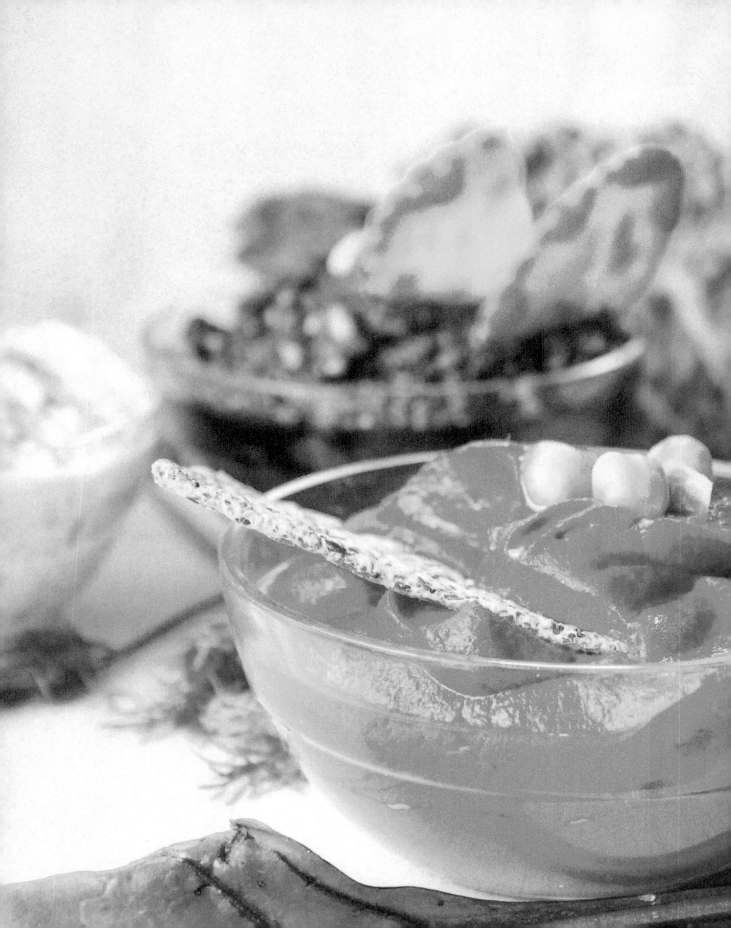

70.   Apple Cider Dressing

Preparation Time: 5 minutes

Cooking time: 0 minutes

Servings: 2

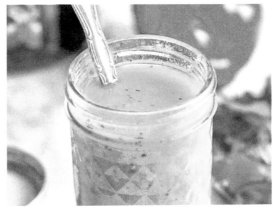

Ingredients:

- 2 tbsps. apple cider vinegar
- 1/3 lemon, juiced
- 1/3 lemon, zested
- Salt, and freshly ground black pepper, to taste

Directions:

1. In a jar, combine the vinegar, lemon juice, and zest. Season with salt, and pepper, cover, and shake well.
2. Use to dress salads or vegetables. Store in the refrigerator.

CHAPTER 9

Nutrition:

Calories: 4   Carbs: 1g

71.   Arugula Walnut Pesto

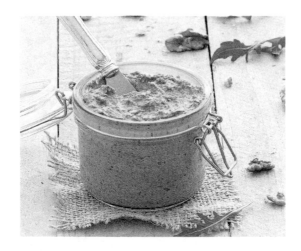

Preparation Time: 5 minutes

Cooking time: 0 minutes

Servings: 8

Ingredients:
- 6 cups packed arugula
- 1 cup chopped walnuts
- ½ cup shredded Parmesan cheese
- 2 garlic cloves, peeled
- ½ tsp salt
- 1 cup extra-virgin olive oil

Directions:
1. In a food processor, combine the arugula, walnuts, cheese, and garlic, and blend until smooth. Add the salt, and, with the processor running, add the olive oil in a drizzle until well blended.
2. Store in a sealed container in the refrigerator.
3. Note: At the time of use, if the mixture seems too thick, add 1 tbsp. of hot water at a time until smooth, and creamy.

Nutrition:

Calories: 296   Fat: 31g   Protein: 4g   Fiber: 1 g
Carbs: 2g

72. Avocado Dip

Preparation Time: 5 minutes
Cooking time: 0 minutes
Servings: 8

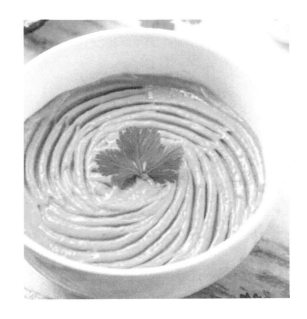

Ingredients:

- ½ cup heavy cream
- 1 green chili pepper, chopped
- Salt, and pepper to the taste
- 4 avocados, pitted, peeled, and chopped
- 1 cup cilantro, chopped
- ¼ cup lime juice

Directions:

1. In a food processor, combine all ingredients, and blend until smooth, and homogeneous.
2. Divide the mix into bowls and serve cold as a dip.

Nutrition:

Calories: 200   Fat: 14.5g   Protein: 7.6g   Fiber: 3.8g
Carbs: 8.1 g

73. Avocado, Cilantro, and White Bean Dip

Preparation Time: 10 minutes

Cooking time: 5 minutes

Servings: 6

Ingredients:

- 15 oz. cannellini beans
- 1 large ripe avocado
- 2 tbsp sour cream
- 2 tbsp Jalapeno slices
- 2 garlic cloves
- ½ cup fresh spinach
- 2-3 tbsp fresh lime juice
- 2 tbsp fresh cilantro plus extra to taste
- 2 tbsp olive oil plus extra to garnish
- ½ tsp ground cumin
- ¼ tsp salt

Directions:

1. In a food processor, place all sauce ingredients, and blend until smooth.
2. Store in the refrigerator until ready to use.
3. If desired, garnish with sliced cherry tomatoes, cilantro, and red onions.
4. Serve with vegetables, corn tortilla chips, flax seeds, crackers, or pita bread

Nutrition:

Calories: 144   Carbs: 18g   Fat: 5g   Protein: 6g

74. Bagna Cauda

Preparation Time: 5 minutes

Cooking time: 20 minutes

Servings: 8

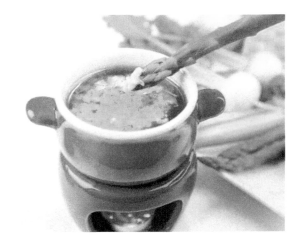

Ingredients:
- ½ cup extra-virgin olive oil
- 4 tbsps. (½ stick)
- 8 anchovy fillets, very finely chopped
- 4 large garlic cloves, finely minced
- ½ tsp salt
- ½ tsp freshly ground black pepper

Directions:
1. In a small saucepan, heat the olive oil, and butter over medium-low heat.
2. When the butter is melted, add the anchovies, and garlic, and stir to combine.
3. Add the salt, and pepper, and reduce the heat to low. Cook, stirring occasionally until the anchovies are very soft, and the mixture is very fragrant about 15-20 minutes.
4. Store in an airtight container in the refrigerator for up to 2 weeks.
5. Serve hot over steamed vegetables, as a dipping sauce for raw vegetables or cooked artichokes, or as a salad dressing

Nutrition:

Calories: 181   Carbs: 1g   Fat: 20g   Protein: 1g

75.   Chickpea, Parsley, and Dill Dip

Preparation Time: 1 night

Cooking time: 2 hours

Servings: 6

Ingredients:

- 1 cup dried chickpeas
- 3 tbsps. olive oil
- 2 garlic cloves
- 2 tbsps. fresh parsley
- 2 tbsps. fresh dill
- 1 tbsp. lemon juice
- ¼ tsp salt

Directions:

1. Soak the chickpeas overnight.
2. In a saucepan, add 1 tbsp. of oil, the water, and the chickpeas, and cook covered for 2 hours.
3. Drain the chickpeas and place them in a food processor along with the garlic, parsley, dill, lemon juice, and the remaining 2 tbsps. of water. Blend for about 30 seconds.
4. With the processor running, slowly add the remaining 2 tbsps. oil, and salt.
5. Serve warm or at room temperature

Nutrition:

Calories: 76   Fat: 4g   Protein: 2g

76. Cocktail Sauce

Preparation Time: 10 minutes

Cooking time: 0 minutes

Servings: 3

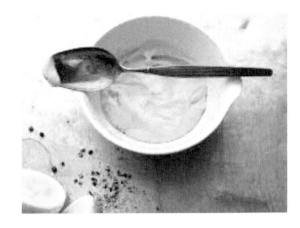

Ingredients:

- 1 tbsp. Worcestershire sauce
- 1 tsp Cognac
- 1 tbsp Mustard
- 2 tbsps. Ketchup
- 7oz mayonnaise

Directions:

1. In a bowl, mix the mayonnaise, and ketchup. Add one tbsp. of mustard, and one tbsp. of Worcestershire sauce, and mix until smooth. Add the cognac and mix until smooth.
2. Place the cocktail sauce in the refrigerator for half an hour, then serve it paired with your dishes.

Nutrition:

Calories: 676   Carbs: 5g   Fat: 10g   Protein: 2.1g

77. Creamy Cucumber Sauce

Preparation Time: 10 minutes

Cooking time: 0 minutes

Servings: 6

Ingredients:
- 1 medium cucumber, peeled, and grated
- ¼ tsp salt
- 1 cup plain Greek yogurt
- 2 garlic cloves, minced
- 1 tbsp. extra-virgin olive oil
- 1 tbsp. freshly squeezed lemon juice
- ¼ tsp freshly ground black pepper

Directions:
1. Place grated cucumber in a strainer over a bowl, and salt. Allow cucumber to stand for 10 minutes. Wrap the cucumber in a cotton cloth and squeeze out as much liquid as possible.
2. Transfer the grated cucumber to a medium bowl. Add the yogurt, garlic, olive oil, lemon juice, and pepper, and mix until well combined. Cover the bowl with plastic wrap and let sit in the refrigerator for at least 2 hours. Serve chilled.

Nutrition:

Calories: 47   Carbs: 2.7g   Fat: 2.8g   Protein: 4.2g

78.   Cucumber Yogurt Dip

Preparation Time: 5 minutes

Cooking time: 0 minutes

Servings: 2

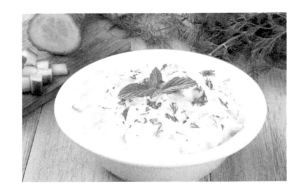

Ingredients:

- 1 cup plain, unsweetened, full-fat Greek yogurt
- ½ cup cucumber, peeled, seeded, and diced 1 tbsp. freshly squeezed lemon juice
- 1 tbsp. chopped fresh mint
- 1 small garlic clove, minced
- Salt, and freshly ground black pepper, to taste

Directions:

1. In a food processor, combine yogurt, cucumber, lemon juice, mint, and garlic.
2. Pulse several times but leave cucumber pieces behind. Season with salt, and pepper, and let sit in the refrigerator until ready to use.

Nutrition:

Calories: 128   Carbs: 7g   Fat: 6g   Protein: 11g

79. Creamy Yogurt Dressing

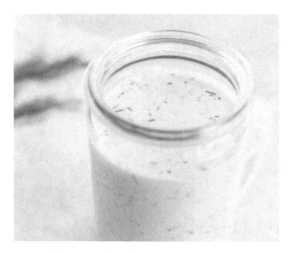

Preparation Time: 5 minutes

Cooking time: 0 minutes

Servings: 3

Ingredients:

- 1 cup plain, unsweetened, full-fat Greek yogurt
- ½ cup extra-virgin olive oil
- 1 tbsp. apple cider vinegar
- ½ lemon, juiced
- 1 tbsp. chopped fresh oregano
- ½ tsp. parsley, chopped
- ½ tsp kosher salt
- ¼ tsp garlic powder
- ¼ tsp freshly ground black pepper

Directions:

1. In a large bowl, combine the yogurt, olive oil, vinegar, lemon juice, oregano, parsley, salt, garlic powder, and pepper, and whisk well. Keep refrigerated until ready to use.

Nutrition:

Calories: 402   Carbs: 4g   Fat: 40g   Protein: 8g

80. Eggplant Pesto

Preparation Time: 10 minutes

Cooking time: 1 hour

Servings: 3

Ingredients:

- 2.2 pounds Eggplants
- 2 oz. pine nuts
- 3 ½ tbsps. Grated Grana Padano
- ¼ cup of extra virgin olive oil
- Min, salt, and pepper to taste

Directions:

1. Preheat the oven to 425°F and line a baking sheet with baking paper.
2. Wash, and dry the eggplants, place them on the lined baking sheet, and pierce them with the ends of a fork. Bake in the oven for 45-50 minutes.
3. Let the eggplants cool, then remove the top end, cut them in half, and scoop out the pulp.
4. Place a colander over a bowl. Place the eggplant pulp in the strainer and press down with a fork to remove excess water. Transfer the eggplant pulp to a blender; add the pine nuts, grated Parmesan cheese, extra virgin olive oil, salt, and pepper, and blend for about a minute, until you have a thick, and creamy puree. Finally, add the chopped mint leaves, and mix.
5. Store in the refrigerator until ready to use.

Nutrition:

Calories: 257   Carbs: 8g   Fat: 21.4g   Protein: 8g

81. Feta Artichoke Dip

Preparation Time: 10 minutes

Cooking time: 30 minutes

Servings: 8

Ingredients:

- 8 ounces artichoke hearts, drained and quartered
- ¾ cup basil, chopped
- ¾ cup green olives, pitted and chopped
- 1 cup parmesan cheese, grated
- 5 ounces feta cheese, crumbled

Directions:

1. Preheat the oven to 375°F and line a baking sheet with baking paper.
2. In a food processor, combine the artichokes, basil, and the rest of the ingredients, and blend well.
3. Transfer the mixture to the prepared baking dish and bake for 30 minutes.
4. Transfer to a bowl and serve as a dip.

Nutrition:

Calories: 186   Fat: 12.4g   Protein: 1.5g   Fiber: 0.9g

Carbs: 2.6g

82.   Fresh Herb Butter

Preparation Time: 5 minutes

Cooking time: 0 minutes

Servings: 6

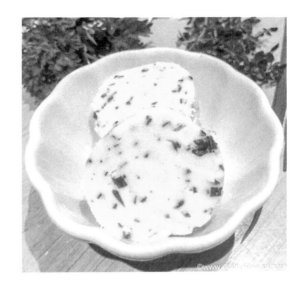

Ingredients:

- ½ cup almond butter, at room temperature
- 1 garlic clove, finely minced
- 2 tsps. finely chopped fresh rosemary
- 1 tsp. finely chopped fresh oregano
- ½ tsp. salt

Directions:

1. In a food processor, combine the almond butter, garlic, rosemary, oregano, and salt, and blend until smooth, and creamy. Transfer the almond butter mixture to a bowl or glass container and refrigerate for up to 1 month.

Nutrition:

Calories: 103   Fat: 12g

83. Genovese Pesto

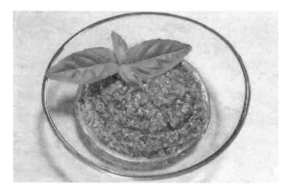

Preparation Time: 20 minutes

Cooking time: 0 minutes

Servings: 2

Ingredients:

- 1 cup(0.9oz) Basil leaves
- 3 ½ tbsp. of extra virgin olive oil
- 2 tbsps. Parmesan cheese to be grated
- 8 tsps. Grated Pecorino
- 1 ½ tbsps. pine nuts
- ½ clove of garlic
- Pinch of coarse salt

Directions:

1. Place the peeled garlic in the mortar along with a few grains of coarse salt, and pound until the garlic is reduced to a paste. Add the basil leaves, and another pinch of coarse salt, and continue to pound by turning the pestle from left to right while simultaneously turning the mortar in the opposite direction.
2. When a bright green liquid comes out of the basil leaves, add the pine nuts, and pound. Add the cheeses a little at a time, stirring constantly, to make the sauce even creamier. Finally, pour in the extra virgin olive oil, continuing to stir with the pestle until the sauce is smooth.
3. Use the pesto as a pasta sauce or on top of a tomato bruschetta

Nutrition:

Calories: 303   Carbs: 1g   Fat: 29g   Protein: 9.5g

84. Ginger Teriyaki Sauce

Preparation Time: 5 minutes
Cooking time: 0 minutes
Servings: 2

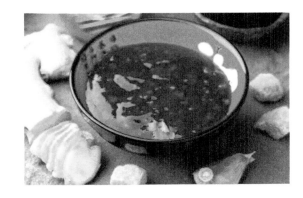

Ingredients:
- ¼ cup pineapple juice
- ¼ cup low-sodium soy sauce
- 2 tbsps. packed coconut sugar
- 1 tbsp. grated fresh ginger
- 1 tbsp. arrowroot powder or cornstarch
- 1 tsp. garlic powder

Directions:
1. In a small bowl, combine the pineapple juice, soy sauce, coconut sugar, ginger, arrowroot powder, and garlic powder, and whisk well with a fork.
2. Store in a wrapped container in the refrigerator for up to 5 days.

Nutrition:

Calories: 37   Carbs: 12g   Fat: 0.1g   Protein: 1.1g

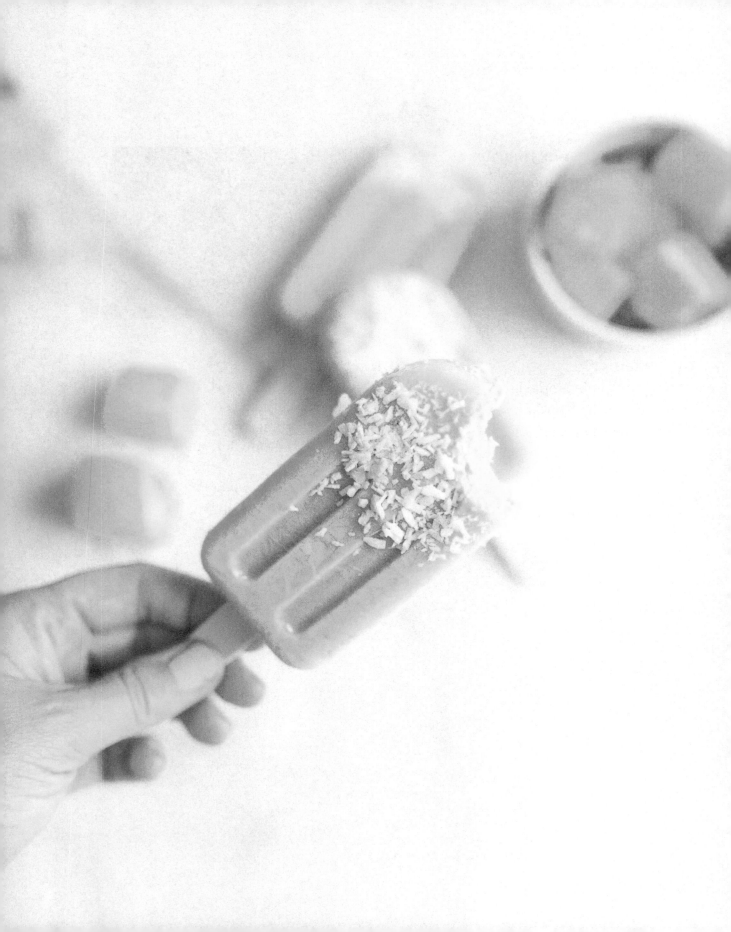

85. Vegan Banana Brownie

Preparation Time: 15 Minutes

Cooking Time: 35 Minutes

Servings: 16 brownies

Ingredients:

- 1 cup of oat flour
- 1 cup of meshed bananas
- ½ cup of cocoa powder
- ½ cup of chopped raw walnuts
- 1/3 cup of unsalted almond butter
- ¼ cup of maple syrup
- 1 tablespoon of dairy-free milk
- 2 teaspoons of vanilla extract
- 1 teaspoon of cinnamon
- 1 teaspoon of baking soda
- ½ teaspoon of sea salt

Directions:

1. Preheat your oven to 350°F. Cover a baking pan with a piece of parchment paper.
2. Mix cocoa powder, oat flour, cinnamon, baking soda, and salt in a mixing bowl. Set aside.
3. Add bananas, almond butter, maple syrup, and vanilla into the other bowl and mix it until well combined.
4. Pour the liquid mixture into the dry one. Add walnuts and stir well to combinate.
5. Spread the batter on the pan and bake for 30–35 minutes until tender.
6. Let it completely cool, then divide into 16 pieces.
7. Serve and enjoy!

Nutrition:

Calories: 122   Fat: 6g   Protein: 3g   Carbohydrates: 17g

CHAPTER 10

86. Oatmeal Cookies

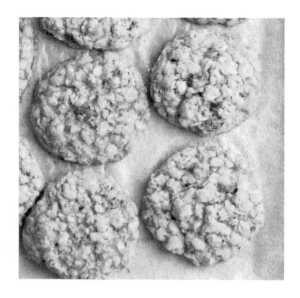

Preparation Time: 10 Minutes

Cooking Time: 15 Minutes

Servings: 12

Ingredients:

- ¼ Cup Applesauce
- ½ Teaspoon Cinnamon
- 1/3 Cup Raisins
- ½ Teaspoon Vanilla Extract, Pure
- 1 Cup Ripe Banana, Mashed
- 2 Cups Oatmeal

Directions:

1. Start by heating your oven to 350.
2. Mix everything together. It should be gooey.
3. Drop it onto an ungreased baking sheet by the tablespoon, and then flatten.
4. Bake for fifteen minutes.

Nutrition:

Calories: 79   Fat: 1g   Protein: 2g   Carbohydrates: 16g

87. Chocolatey Bean Mousse

Preparation Time: 10 Minutes

Cooking Time: 10 Minutes

Servings: 3

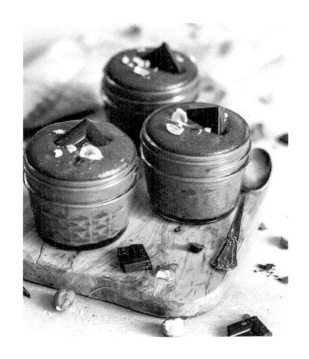

Ingredients:

- ½ cup unsweetened almond milk
- 1 cup cooked black beans
- 4 Medjool dates, pitted and chopped
- ½ cup walnuts, chopped
- 2 tablespoons cacao powder
- 1 teaspoon vanilla extract
- 3 tablespoons fresh blueberries
- 1 teaspoon fresh mint leaves

Directions:

1. In a food processor, add all ingredients and pulse until smooth and creamy.
2. Transfer the mousse into serving bowls and refrigerate to chill before serving.
3. Garnish with blueberries and mint leaves and serve.

Nutrition:

Calories: 465   Fat: 14g   Protein: 21g;   Carbohydrates: 70g

88. Tofu and Strawberry Mousse

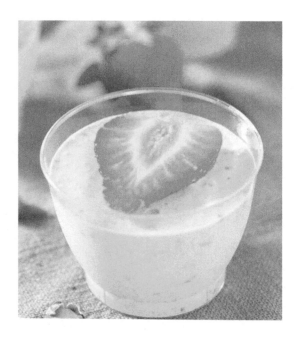

Preparation Time: 10 Minutes

Cooking Time: 10 Minutes

Servings: 4

Ingredients:

- 2 cups fresh strawberries, hulled and sliced
- 2 cups firm tofu, pressed and drained
- 3 tablespoons maple syrup
- 4 tablespoons walnuts, chopped

Directions:

1. In a blender, add the strawberries and pulse until just pureed.
2. Add the tofu and maple syrup and pulse until smooth.
3. Transfer the mousse into serving bowls and refrigerate to chill before serving.
4. Garnish with walnuts and serve.

Nutrition:

Calories: 199   Fat: 10g   Carbohydrates: 18g   Protein: 13g

89.   Tofu and Chia Seed Pudding

Preparation Time: 15 Minutes

Cooking Time: 15 Minutes

Servings: 4

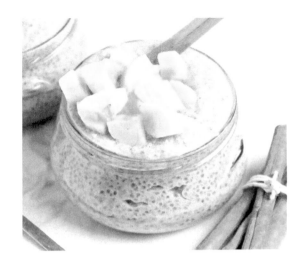

Ingredients:
- 1-pound silken tofu, pressed and drained
- ¼ cup banana, peeled
- 3 tablespoons cacao powder
- 1 teaspoon vanilla extract
- 3 tablespoons chia seeds
- ¼ cup walnuts, chopped

¼ cup black raisins

Directions:
1. In a food processor, add tofu, banana, cocoa powder, and vanilla, and pulse till smooth and creamy.
2. Transfer into a large serving bowl and stir in chia seeds till well mixed.
3. Now, place the pudding in serving bowls evenly.
4. With plastic wraps, cover the bowls. Refrigerate to chill before serving.
5. Garnish with raspberries and serve

Nutrition:

Calories: 188   Fat: 10g   Carbohydrates: 17g   Protein: 12g

90. Brown Rice Pudding

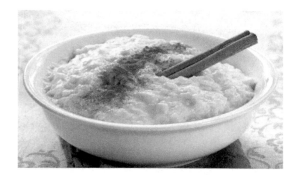

Preparation Time: 15 Minutes

Cooking Time: 1 Hour 15 Minutes

Servings: 2

Ingredients:

- ½ cup brown basmati rice, soaked for 15 minutes and drained 1½ cups water
- 2½ cups unsweetened almond milk
- 4 tablespoons cashews
- 2–3 tablespoons maple syrup
- 1/8 teaspoon ground cardamom
- Pinch of salt
- 3 tablespoons golden raisins
- 2 tablespoons cashews
- 2 tablespoons almonds

Directions:

1. In a pan, add the rice and water over medium-high heat and bring to a boil.
2. Lower the heat to medium and cook for about 30 minutes.
3. Meanwhile, in a blender, add the almond milk and cashews and pulse until smooth.
4. In the pan of rice, slowly add the milk mixture stirring continuously.
5. Sir in the maple syrup, cardamom, and salt, and cook for about 15–20 minutes, stirring occasionally.
6. Stir in the raisins and cook for about 15–20 minutes, stirring occasionally.
7. Remove from the heat and set aside to cool slightly.
8. Serve warm with the garnishing of banana slices and pistachios.

Nutrition :

Calories: 498   Protein: 11g   Carbohydrates: 73g   Fats: 21g

Chapter 11: 4 Weeks Meal-Plan

Day	Breakfast	Lunch	Snack	Dinner
1	Quinoa black beans breakfast bowl	Split pea pesto stuffed shells	Mango and banana shake	Romaine lettuce and radicchios mix
2	Corn griddle cakes with tofu mayonnaise	Coriander okra and kale	Avocado toast with flaxseeds	Greek salad
3	Savory breakfast salad	Thai peanut and sweet potato buddha bowl	Plant-based crispy falafel	Roasted pepper pasta salad
4	Almond plum oats overnight	Buffalo cauliflower tacos	Almond plum oats overnight	Salad Niçoise
5	High protein: toast	Peanut vegetable noodle bowl	Simple banana fritters	Tomato salad
6	Hummus carrot sandwich	Pumpkin penne	Coconut and blueberries ice cream	Cauliflower sweet potato salad
7	Overnight oats	White bean and mushroom meatballs subs	Avocado chat	Cauliflower sweet potato salad
8	Avocado miso chickpeas toast	White bean and mushroom meatballs subs	Crispy brinjal "bacon"	Tropical style Radicchio salad
9	Banana vegan bread	Sweet potato fries	Pomegranate flower sprouts	Winter vegetable salad
10	Banana malt bread	Zucchini soup	Banana curry	Vegan cobb salad
11	Quinoa black beans breakfast bowl	Vegetarian Biryani	Mushroom curry	Greek-style spring soup
12	Avocado miso chickpeas toast	Roasted cauliflower	Veggie combo	Coconut lemon lentil soup
13	High protein: toast	Chinese eggplant with Szechuan sauce	Squash black bean bowl	Apple and butternut squash soup
14	Quinoa black beans breakfast bowl	Ramen with miso shiitake	Vegan banana brownie	Quinoa vegetable soup
15	Overnight oats	Butternut squash linguine	Oatmeal cookies	Cauliflower and horseradish soup
16	Banana malt bread	Sweet potato and bean burgers	Chocolatey bean mousse	Chickpea noodle soup

17	Banana vegan bread	Thai peanut sauce over roasted sweet potatoes	Tofu and strawberry mousse	Cauliflower sweet potato salad
18	Avocado miso chickpeas toast	Burrito-stuffed sweet potatoes	Tofu and chia seed pudding	Apple and butternut squash soup
19	Banana malt bread	Butternut squash chipotle chili	Brown rice pudding	Cauliflower sweet potato salad
20	High protein: toast	Winter vegetable salad	Almond butter fudge	Quinoa vegetable soup
21	Overnight oats	Tropical style radicchio salad	Almond butter cookies	Roasted pepper pasta salad
22	Quinoa black beans breakfast bowl	Eggplant pesto	Cashew pudding	Apple and butternut squash soup
23	Corn griddle cakes with tofu mayonnaise	Cauliflower sweet potato salad	Peach cobbler	Quinoa vegetable soup
24	Savory breakfast salad	Butternut squash linguine	Black bean orange mousse	Curry lentil soup
25	Almond plum oats overnight	Tomato salad	Almond and chocolate chip bars	Chickpea noodle soup
26	Hummus carrot sandwich	Roasted pepper pasta salad	Mocha fudge	Creamy mushroom soup
27	Overnight oats	Thai peanut sauce over roasted sweet potatoes	Chocolate with coconut and raisins	Tuscany vegetable soup
28	High protein: toast	Burrito-stuffed sweet potatoes	Ice cream	Cabbage soup
29	Corn griddle cakes with tofu mayonnaise	Greek salad	Peach cobbler	Zucchini soup
30	Hummus carrot sandwich	Romaine lettuce and radicchios mix	Cinnamon coconut chips	Roasted red pepper and tomato soup

PBWF Join I.F.

Every day, more people are opting for of PBWF diets, finally, it's becoming the new standard for human health. This is amazing news for those who understand and believe in long term well-being. It's important to note that it's not enough to follow a healthy diet plan without also considering a proper daily training plan to achieve s light and tonic body.

I.F. is one the oldest and working methods to heal human body and brain from the external environment and food toxins. Through the fasting window our body starts to clean itself automatically (**autophagy**) and after almost 30 days all the benefits in term of lightness and more focus comes out.

Skipping a meal, eating one meal a day, or eating in certain time windows can be done with a plant-based diet too. This will further the benefits towards general wellness. Studies on Intermittent Fasting were found likely to have the same beneficial effects on health and longevity as people following a traditional low-calorie diet plan without training.

I.F. Eating Window

To lose weight and clear the brain, would be recommended to eat PBWF and work out more. However, this is hard for people who has the bad habit to assume a lot of calories and does not know the miraculous benefit of daily walking.

Many people don't realize that many will reach their breaking point when they're no longer able to control their appetite during the I.F. Eating Window. At this point, the person will start binging on junk food or foods high in calories that are easy to acquire quickly to get those much-needed calories in.

This is where The I.F. Eating Window comes in. It's a 24-hour time each day where the person can eat as much food as they want as long as it's within the I.F. Eating Window timeframe that they set up (usually lasts for 8 hours).

This gives them a daily calorie allotment that they can use to eat whatever they want within that 24-hour period, which includes all their junk food cravings and calorie-rich foods they've been missing out on.

The rest of the day when the I.F. Eating Window is closed, the person has to stick with eating only until their next I.F. Eating Window opens.

After your first meal, there will be a window of time in which you are going to eat your meals before fasting again. During this window, you can eat as often or as little as you like. Be aware that you want to begin setting yourself up for your next fast near the end of your eating window, so eating your last meal right before the end of this window is advised, to give you better footing and making sure you are ready to fast.

You can use this window however you like—eating two meals or four, for example. How you decide to eat in your eating window will also depend on the way that you have split your fasting and eating—whether over days of the week or hours of the day. This is the part of fasting with the most flexibility, so feel free to experiment with your meals here to see what works the best for your body.

The 16:8 diet

The 16:8 diet is a way of eating with a day of fasting followed by an eighth of the total calories for the rest of the day. This diet can be applied to any style of eating and has been seen as an easier method than other Intermittent Fasting methods such as 5:2, OMAD & EAT stop EAT.

How does it work?

Simply put, you are going to fast for sixteen hours at night and then eat whatever you want for eight hours during the day (most people choose breakfast).

That's it! There are also variations where you can choose what time to fast which would make this easier if you have chronic night shifts. You will have to try this out and see how it works for you as everyone's body is different.

A note on calories: People who are following a strict diet will need to adapt their calorie intake accordingly. Most people find they are consuming 200-400 fewer calories per day which can be easily adjusted through altering the food budget each day. On rare occasions, people may want to increase their calories, but would not want the extra amount of fat or carbohydrates to exceed 2% of the daily calorie intake. Extra nutrients such as vitamins and minerals do not count towards the 1% daily allowance of calories so should be taken with supplements.

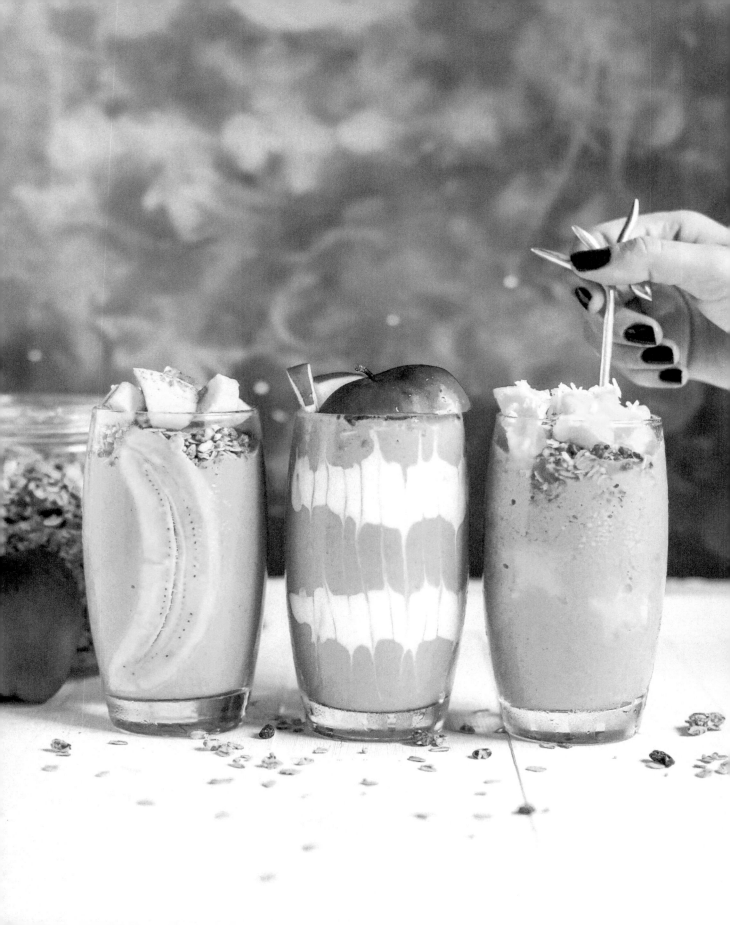

CHAPTER II

Chapter 12: Drinks Giving

Herbal based drinks are and have been a human's favorite since ancient times. It is a simple and clever way to heal disorders and refill fluids lost through the daily activities, like, working, walking, running, shopping...etc. Herbal drinks made from botanical sources are better known as "**infusions**". Infusions are able to pull out all water-soluble wealthy herb properties such as minerals, vitamins, enzymes and proteins well known for their deep cellular level hydration, improve digestion, regulate the immune system, and contain antioxidants. These infusions are worth considering as part of our heathy daily habits.

When the air temperature is cold the human' body naturally loses heat through radiation and conduction of the outdoor environment. This loss of heat will make the body temperature drop, which is the reason why people feel colder and sicker in the winter season. While drinking a hot drink, the gut absorbs the active principles and some heat and transfers it to whole body. Better is the warmup in term of quality drinking, better are the human psychophysical performances and recovery.

Natural herbal infusions play a key role to heal and reverse several human troubles and inflammations, of course is fundamental know exactly the illness symptoms to benefit the equivalent natural herb remedy. Prevention illness is another evident function that infusion performs in human well-being.

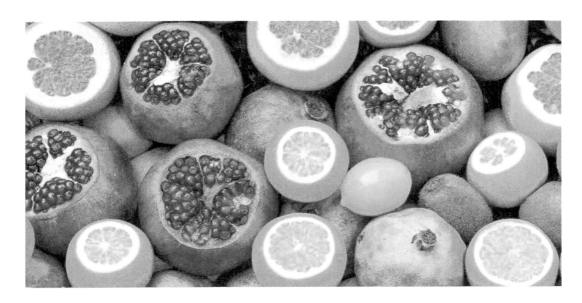

Infusions & tea medicinal properties

Infusions & Tea are drinks that can be enjoyed hot or cold and are largely consumed worldwide, mostly as social drink or just to warm up, without knowing the exact power of them. Powerful antioxidants infusion content, it has been shown to secure significant health benefits. Green drinks have been gaining popularity among health communities because it offers unique health advantages, such as benefiting our **gut** microbiome by providing probiotics for your small intestine that assure better digestion from the inside out

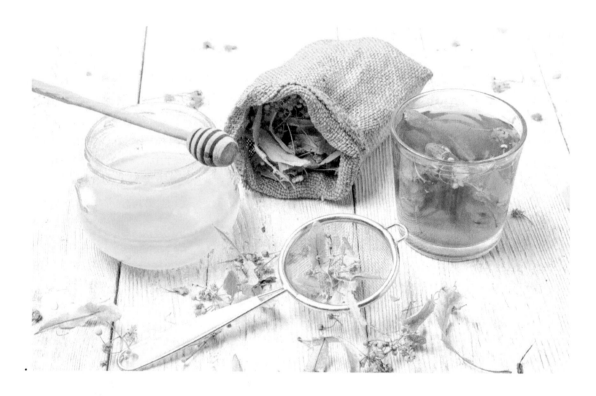

How to brew an infusions or tea...

Selecting the desired flavor profile or mix herbs with spices, soaking tea leaves or herbs in hot water and then, usually, allowing them to steep for 5-8 minutes or even more, to be sure read the labels directions, then enjoy. To brew a healer tasting infusion, you can add spices like cloves, ginger, turmeric, peppermint, which are known to be helpful for general inflammation, better digestion, asthma and respiratory illness.

When creating an infused tea, choose herbs that will work best with personal health goals, for a ginger-infused mint tea, is recommended use fresh organic ginger and organic raw peppermint., to heal flu and breath properly or just to warm up.

...and enjoy healing

- Hydration on a deep, cellular level
- Improved skin texture, turnover, and glow
- Strong, shiny, and fast-growing hair and nails
- Improved digestion
- Mental, emotional, and physical resilience
- Increased energy, focus, and stamina
- Improved hormonal balance
- Immune system regulation (calms an overactive immune system and boosts a sluggish one)

Nourishing dry herbs medicinal list

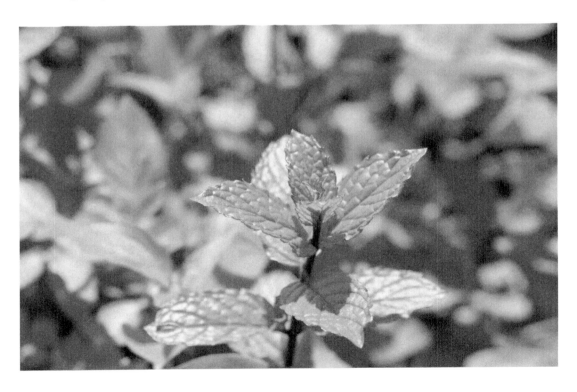

PEPPERMINT (Mentha piperita) high essential oil content helps with cramping, heartburn, gas, and nausea.

RED RASPBERRY (Rubus spp.) woman's tonic herb, ease uterine and intestinal spasms, promoting healthy bones, nails, teeth, and skin

NETTLE (Urtica dioica) overall tonics kidneys, lungs, intestine, arteries, hair, and skin

RED CLOVER (trifolium pratense.) blood purifier and lymphatic mover, help women in menopause, overall skin treatment.

OATSTRAW (oats sativa) anti-depressant and restorative nerve tonic, beneficial lupus, or other autoimmune diseases

HORSETAIL (Equisetum arvense) It improves skin, hair and nails because it helps support healthy connective tissue and collagen.

CALENDULA (Calendula officinalis) anti-inflammatory, antibacterial, antimicrobial, moves **lymph** (detoxification). It helps soothe and heal the gut, helps drain.

HAWTHORNE (Crataegus) general cardiovascular tonic, powerful antioxidants and polyphenols inhibit cholesterol and reduce free radicals

LADY'S MANTLE (Alchemilla vulgaris) amazing female tonic, It helps to ease heavy menstrual flow and cramping with regular use.

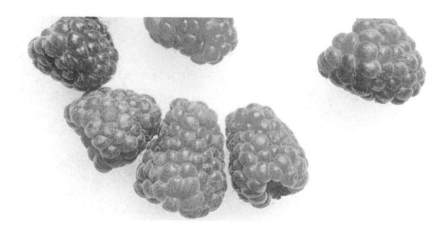

91. Ginger Detox Infusion

Preparation time: 15 minutes

Cooking time: 10 minutes

Servings: 2

Ingredients:
- 1/2 teaspoon of grated ginger, fresh
- 1 small lemon slice
- 1/8 teaspoon of cayenne pepper
- 1/8 teaspoon of ground turmeric
- 1/8 teaspoon of ground cinnamon
- 1 teaspoon of maple syrup
- 1 teaspoon of apple cider vinegar
- 2 cups of boiling water

Directions:
1. Pour the boiling water into a small saucepan, add and stir the ginger, then let it rest for 8 to 10 minutes, before covering the pan.
2. Pass the mixture through a strainer and into the liquid, add the cayenne pepper, turmeric, cinnamon and stir properly.
3. Add the maple syrup, vinegar, and lemon slice.
4. Add and stir an infused lemon and serve immediately.

Nutrition:

Calories:80 Cal   Carbohydrates:0g   Protein:0g   Fiber:0g
Fats:0g

92. Spiced Lemon Drink

Preparation time: 2 hours and 10 mins

Cooking time: 2 hours

Servings: 12

Ingredients:

- 1 cinnamon stick, about 3 inches long
- 1/2 teaspoon of whole cloves
- 2 cups of coconut sugar
- 4 fluid of ounce pineapple juice
- 1/2 cup and 2 tablespoons of lemon juice
- 12 fluid ounce of orange juice
- 2 1/2 quarts of water

Directions:

1. Pour water into a 6-quarts slow cooker and stir the sugar and lemon juice properly.
2. Wrap the cinnamon, the whole cloves in cheesecloth and tie its corners with string.
3. Immerse this cheesecloth bag in the liquid present in the slow cooker and cover it with the lid.
4. Then plug in the slow cooker and let it cook on high heat setting for 2 hours or until it is heated thoroughly.
5. When done, discard the cheesecloth bag and serve the drink hot or cold.

Nutrition:

Calories:15 Cal   Carbohydrates:3.2g   Protein:0.1g   Fiber:0g
Fats:0g

93. Soothing Ginger Tea Drink

Preparation time: 2 hours and 15 mins
Cooking time: 2 hours and 10 minutes
Servings: 8

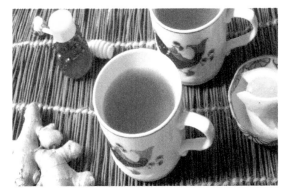

Ingredients:

- 1 tablespoon of minced ginger root
- 2 tablespoons of honey
- 15 green tea bags
- 32 fluid ounce of white grape juice
- 2 quarts of boiling water

Directions:

1. Pour water into a 4-quarts slow cooker, immerse tea bags, cover the cooker and let stand for 10 minutes.
2. After 10 minutes, remove and discard tea bags and stir in remaining ingredients.
3. Return cover to slow cooker, then plug in and let cook at high heat setting for 2 hours or until heated through.
4. When done, strain the liquid and serve hot or cold.

Nutrition:

Calories:45 Cal
Fats:0g
Carbohydrates:12g
Protein:0g
Fiber:0g

94. Tangy Cranberry Infusion

Preparation time: 3 hours and 10 mins

Cooking time: 3 hours

Servings: 14

Ingredients:
- 1 1/2 cups of coconut sugar
- 12 whole cloves
- 2 fluid ounce of lemon juice
- 6 fluid ounce of orange juice
- 32 fluid ounces of cranberry juice
- 8 cups of hot water
- 1/2 cup of Red-Hot candies

Directions:
1. Pour the water into a 6-quarts slow cooker along with the cranberry juice, orange juice, and the lemon juice.
2. Stir the sugar properly.
3. Wrap the whole cloves in a cheese cloth, tie its corners with strings, and immerse it in the liquid present inside the slow cooker.
4. Add the red-hot candies to the slow cooker and cover it with the lid.
5. Then plug in the slow cooker and let it cook on the low heat setting for 3 hours or until it is heated thoroughly.
6. When done, discard the cheesecloth bag and serve.

Nutrition:

Calories:89 Cal   Carbohydrates:27g   Protein:0g   Fiber:1g
Fats:0g

95. Lemony Ginger Tea

Preparation time: 10 minutes
Cooking time: 10 minutes
Servings: 1

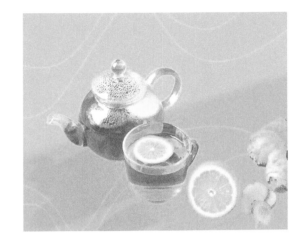

Ingredients:
- 1 teaspoon finely grated fresh ginger root
- 1 cup boiling water
- 1 lemon wedge (about ⅛ of a lemon)

Directions:
1. Place ginger root in a tea infuser and set in mug. Pour water into mug and let steep for about 10 minutes.
2. Remove infuser from tea. Squeeze juice from lemon wedge into tea, sweeten if desired and serve immediately. Enjoy!

Nutrition:

calories: 0   protein: 0g   carbs: 0g   fiber: 0g
fat: 0g   net carbs: 0g

96. Balmy Infusion

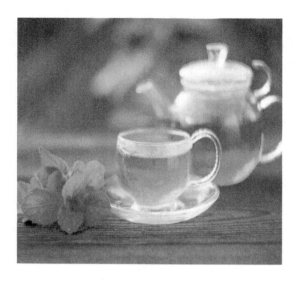

Preparation Time: 5 minutes

Cooking Time: 5 minutes

Servings: 1

Ingredients:

- 1 Tbsp Lemon zest
- 1 Cup Peppermint
- 5 Cup Water

Directions:

1. Set the water up to boil. When it reaches a boil, add in zest and peppermint.
2. Take off the heat and allow it to cool down 15 min. before straining and serving

Nutrition:

Calories: 13.3   Carbohydrates: 3.6 g   Proteins: 1 g   Cholesterol: 0 mg

Fats: 0 g   Sugars: 0 g

97.   Cinnamon Tea

Preparation Time: 1 minute
Cooking Time: 5 minutes
Servings: 1

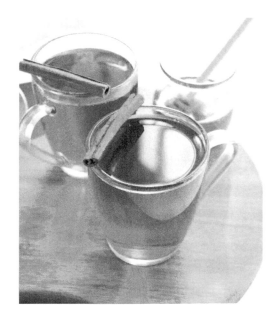

Ingredients:
- 1 Tbsp. Cinnamon
- 1 Cup Water
- 5 Cup Lemon

Directions:
1. Add the water to a pan and bring to boil. Add in the cinnamon and stir to help it dissolve.
2. Squeeze the lemon into the tea and stir well. Serve hot.

Nutrition:

Calories: 9   Carbohydrates: 2.5   Proteins: 0.2 g   Cholesterol: 0 mg
Fats: 0 g   g Sugars: 0.1 g

98. Turmeric Infusion

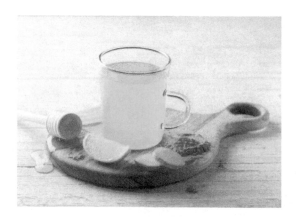

Preparation Time: 1 minute

Cooking Time: 5 minutes

Servings: 1

Ingredients:

- 1 Tbsp. Raw honey
- 2 Cup Water
- ¼ Tbsp Turmeric
- Sage Leaves just enough

Directions:

1. Add the water into a pan and let it heat up to boil. When boiling, take off the heat.
2. Add in the turmeric and sage leaves and let it rest in there for a bit.
3. After 15 minutes, strain the tea and pour it into cups. Stir in pepper and honey and serve hot.

Nutrition:

Calories: 35   Carbohydrates: 8 g   Proteins: 0.1 g   Cholesterol: 0 mg
Fats: 0 g   Sugars: 0 g

99. Basil Infusion

Preparation Time: 5 minutes
Cooking Time: 30 minutes
Servings: 1

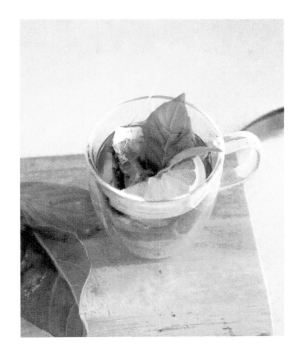

Ingredients:

- Honey (1 tsp.)
- Water (1 c.)
- Fresh Basil Leaves just enough
- ½ Lemon juice & zest

Directions:

1. Add your lemon juice and zest to some boiling water and let it rest there for 30 minutes.
2. When that time is up, strain it out and add basil and honey. Stir well and serve it nice and hot.

Nutrition:

Calories 20	Carbs 4g	Fat 0g	Protein 0.1g

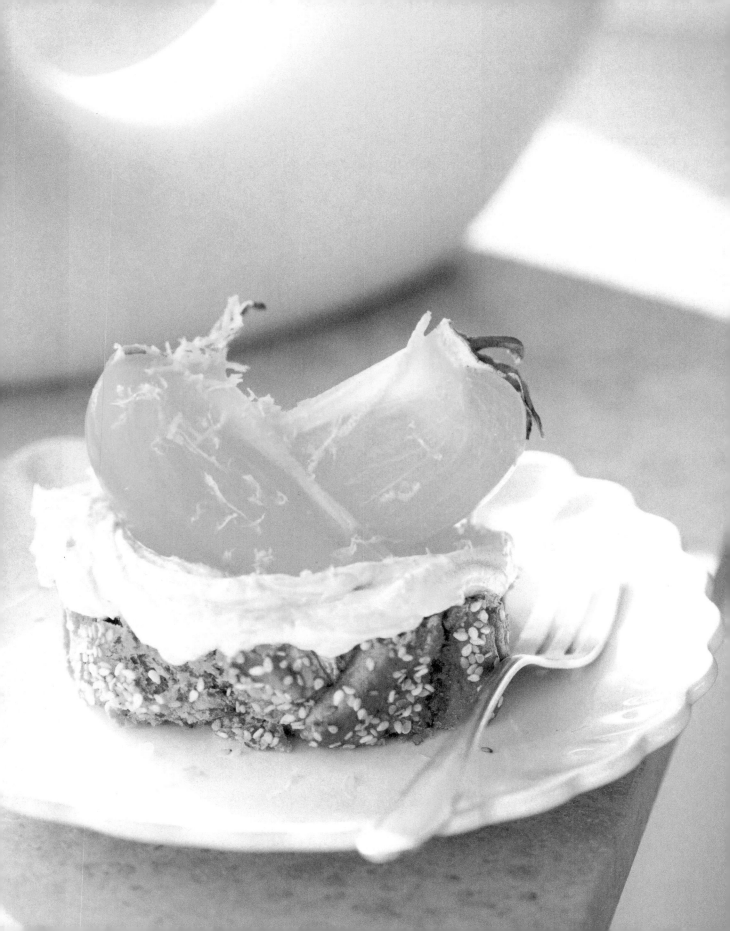

Conclusion

Plant-based eating method warmly suggests excluding any animal based, processed and refined food from our daily diet.

Studies claim that the human body should be more alkaline than acidic. An acidic diet is not expected for optimum health. The key to healthy living starts with a de-acidifying diet, then rich in vegetables, organic plant-based proteins, low carbs, and whole food.

With vegetables proteins in your diet, your body will gradually be re-balanced to an alkaline state. Alkalinity helps prevent and reverse: blood and joint inflammations, diabetes type 2-3, arthritis, psoriasis, and several contemporary diseases. Plant eating are high in water and low in sugar - therefore they have a low glycemic load, studies have been shown to have anti-inflammatory properties and contain a multitude of highly nutritious phytonutrients, vitamins, and minerals that make them much healthier nutritious than animal-based food.

Vegetables are filled with powerful antioxidants such as beta carotene, lutein, zeaxanthin, vitamin C, vitamin E, and flavonoids. These antioxidants help protect and reverse the body from diseases and they play a vital role in protecting all cells throughout the body - by combatting free radicals which are believed to be the cause of many modern diseases.

The high-water content of vegetables and the significant levels of fiber in whole grains food, make them naturally low in calories, and amazing in perfect gut & kidneys performances.

The alkaline PH of vegetables is pH 7 compared to a body pH that is slightly acidic on average at around PH 7.4 - this is important when considering how your body performs in comparison to an environment with more food acidity.

Blood tests can give an important information about the pH and mineral content of bodily fluids not normally tested by doctors. It is proved that cancer cells thrive in an acid environment - so here is one example of how an alkaline diet help prevent many kinds of cancer.

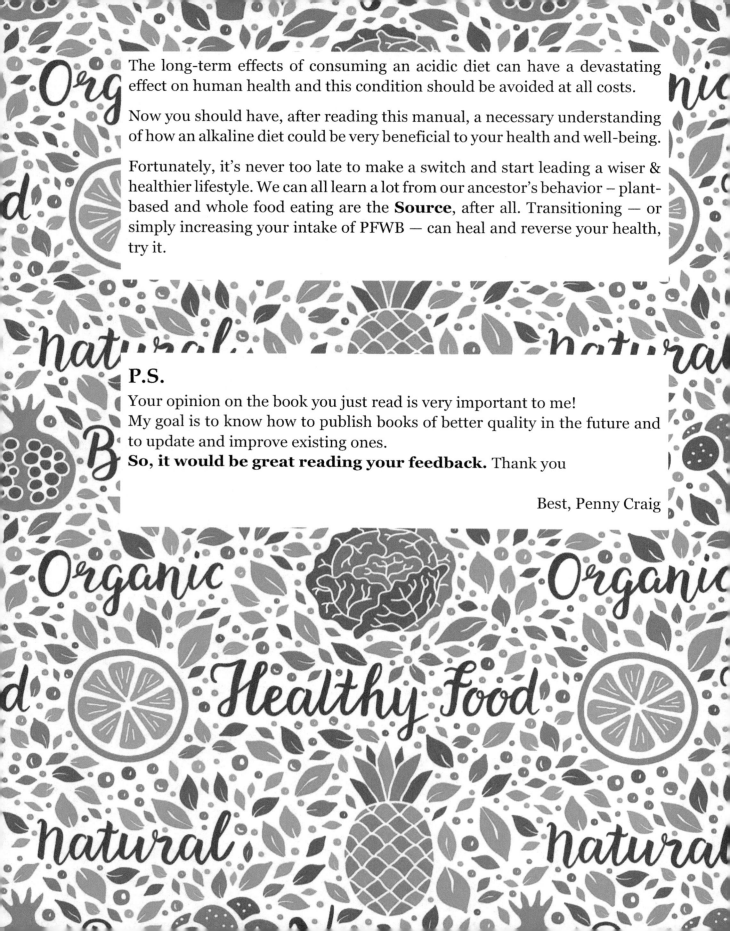

The long-term effects of consuming an acidic diet can have a devastating effect on human health and this condition should be avoided at all costs.

Now you should have, after reading this manual, a necessary understanding of how an alkaline diet could be very beneficial to your health and well-being.

Fortunately, it's never too late to make a switch and start leading a wiser & healthier lifestyle. We can all learn a lot from our ancestor's behavior – plant-based and whole food eating are the **Source**, after all. Transitioning — or simply increasing your intake of PFWB — can heal and reverse your health, try it.

P.S.

Your opinion on the book you just read is very important to me!
My goal is to know how to publish books of better quality in the future and to update and improve existing ones.
So, it would be great reading your feedback. Thank you

Best, Penny Craig